CHIA SEED REMEDIES

CHIA SEED
REMEDIES

USE THESE ANCIENT SEEDS TO:
LOSE WEIGHT • BALANCE BLOOD SUGAR
FEEL ENERGIZED • SLOW AGING
DECREASE INFLAMMATION
AND MORE!

MySeeds Chia Test Kitchen

Skyhorse Publishing

Skyhorse Publishing books may be purchased in bulk at special discounts for sales promotion, corporate gifts, fund-raising, or educational purposes. Special editions can also be created to specifications. For details, contact the Special Sales Department, Skyhorse Publishing, 307 West 36th Street, 11th Floor, New York, NY 10018 or info@skyhorsepublishing.com.

Skyhorse® and Skyhorse Publishing® are registered trademarks of Skyhorse Publishing, Inc.®, a Delaware corporation.

Visit our website at www.skyhorsepublishing.com.

10 9 8 7 6 5 4 3

Library of Congress Cataloging-in-Publication Data

MySeeds Chia Test Kitchen.
Chia seed remedies : Use these ancient seeds to lose weight, balance blood sugar, feel energized, slow aging, decrease inflammation, and more! / by MySeeds Chia Test Kitchen.
    pages cm

ISBN 978-1-62636-391-5 (alk. paper)

1. Chia. 2. Health—Nutritional aspects. 3. Cooking (Seeds) 4. Cooking (Natural foods) I. Title.

TX558.C38C63 2012
641.6'56—dc23

                                    2013031842

Printed in the United States of America

CONTENTS

• • • • • • • • •

INTRODUCTION

The MySeeds kitchen is comprised of "sunny-side-up" people who love whole natural foods. We love science and the ecosystem of the human body. We feel that life should be interesting, fun, lively, and tasty and that incorporating foods like chia into our lives helps us live more fully. With a little planning and thought, we know that chia seeds will enhance your life too. Chia has so many health benefits that we just had to spread the word about it. This book is a compilation of research from a variety of scientific sources combined with a good dose of plain common sense. We hope the thoughts and recipes we offer will help you understand how to make your body healthier and happier and how to give yourself more energy to have more *fun*. Sound good? Let's get started!

NOTICE:

The statements in this book are reflective of the authors' experiences. Yours may be different. As always, you should consult with your physician before making changes to your diet or taking supplements. Chia is not intended to prevent, treat, cure, or diagnose any disease. We feel, as so many people do, that including chia in our eating habits has enhanced our lives.

WARNING:

Chia seeds are not "magical" seeds. They cannot be sprinkled onto or into your food and then magically transform your body into the person you want to be. They're not a pharmaceutical pill you can take to rev your metabolism or suddenly experience a blast of artificial energy. Chia provides nutrients your body needs, as well as fiber and protein for steady, non-jittery energy.

There's a lot of hype surrounding chia seeds today. Some companies are trying to genetically modify certain chia plants for patents, while others are using multilevel marketing schemes to sell the seeds, which can lead to some outlandish claims. It's important to do research for yourself and get the real facts so that you can avoid being swept up in the hype of a "new" food. Chia is actually ancient but is currently experiencing a well-deserved return to the spotlight as health enthusiasts rediscover this fantastic seed.

However, chia seeds added to a healthy eating lifestyle can help you transform your body into a healthier you. Chia seeds are packed with so many vital minerals, nutrients, and omega-3 fats that you are most likely missing from your diet. They will help you control your appetite and sugar levels. Chia will keep you hydrated for energy and endurance. But chia is not magical, it just may seem a bit magical once you learn how to up your nutrition by using these little seeds.

A LITTLE BIT ON HEALTHY EATING:

We bet you are thinking, how hard is this healthy lifestyle going to be? How much tasteless "tofu-ish" food can I stand? How much time is this going to take? How can I get my act together and accomplish this new proposition? How hard is the chia seed to use? Well, it is easy! We will show you how easy, fast, and fun it can be. (We are not really tofu fans, by the way.) You already do a lot of food preparation that is smart. You broil or bake a chicken. You do eat fish. You do serve veggies. You do make salads. Let's just up your game!

We have included many chia recipes that we are certain you will enjoy and are *fast* and *easy*. Because chia seeds are flavorless, you can't hate them, but they could get boring (no taste = no fun) if you don't have creative ways to use these healthy seeds. Each recipe illustrates a point in the book. For example, if you're looking to help your picky-eating kids get better nutrition, there are chia recipes to help you. If your goal is to have a meatless night in a house full of carnivores, you can find some recipes that everyone may agree on. This book is here to help you implement any or all of the healthy advice with examples and recipes that anyone can do.

You can use some of *your* favorite recipes and perhaps tweak them and add chia to up your fullness factor and add nutrition. To make planning meals easier, we started by making a list of all the dinners and lunches the whole family liked. Just ask around the dinner table before your designated grocery day, "What sounds good for the next week or the next few days?" I'm sure you will get suggestions that everyone will agree on. Now, gather up the recipes and see what fill-ins or other ingredients you will require. Ta-da! Your list is close to being complete.

A few of the recipes are sides. These are meant to accompany a piece of meat or fish. These sides would replace the mac and cheese, the instant mashed potato pile, the oven-baked frozen french fries. You want a pizza? We have one. You would like a burger? We have one (actually, lots of them). You want easy ideas for a taco salad? Would you like a few easy salad dressings too? OK, it is just that fast. You'll be so surprised at the super variety of recipes that you can make easily with chia seeds. Let's get started!

What Is the Chia Seed?

Chia seeds are tiny seeds that come from the *Salvia hispanica* plant. This plant is a relative of the mint family. It's a hardy plant that grows in sandy or rocky soil in hot, dry regions. It originated in the high-altitude desert area of Mexico. It's believed to have gotten started in the Chiapas region, which gave it the modern name of "chia."[1]

Chia is actually much older than many people know. It has been used since the time of the ancient Aztecs. Chia seeds were prized by ancient people because of their nutrition and hunger-fighting properties. These lightweight seeds could help soldiers travel for longer periods without food. The Tarahumara natives (a more recent people than the Aztecs) call chia "the running food" and are known for consuming it on their amazing marathons through harsh desert conditions.[2] Chia has a long, safe, and productive history of being used by humankind.[3]

Chia seeds come in two colors, mostly black and mostly white. Neither one has any flavor. That's the first great property of chia. Because it has no taste, no one can hate it! Chia is tiny, about the size of a poppy seed. Often, if you're eating chia, you won't even notice. That's what helps make it so great: you can add a healthy boost to almost any food you already like to eat by adding chia. You won't taste the difference, but your body will know, as chia adds nutrients, fiber, and protein.

---

1 Wikipedia, "Salvia Hispanica," http://en.wikipedia.org/wiki/Salvia_hispanica (Accessed 22 October 2013)

2 *Ultra Running*, "Chia Seeds The Running Food," http://ultrarunning.co.nz/content/chia-seeds-running-food (Accessed 22 October 2013)

3 Dr. Brent Agin and Shereen Jegtvig, *Superfoods for Dummies*, (Wily Publishing Inc. 2009), 154

What's in These Seeds?

There are so many great aspects of chia that you could write a book about them all! And, in fact, you are holding that book right now. We'll elaborate on each of these aspects with examples, recipes, charts, and more.

1. Chia has complete protein like that found in meat, but it is a 100 percent plant product. That's not all that common in the edible plant world.

2. Chia has two kinds of fiber: soluble and insoluble. The insoluble fiber is what you see as the seed shell. This type of fiber can't be digested. It acts as a sweeper, helping move food through the digestive system smoothly and efficiently. The soluble fiber can be seen only if you create chia gel. It's on the outside of the seed shell, and it can hold onto nine times its weight in water. This forms a little bead of gel. This type of fiber can't be digested either, but healthy bacteria (flora) of the digestive tract thrive in the presence of soluble fiber. This fiber also helps hydrate the colon for better nutrient absorption.

3. Chia has more calcium by weight than milk.

4. Chia has more magnesium than broccoli. Magnesium is the mineral that can help prevent more than twenty-two different health conditions. It's much more important than people give it credit for, so be sure to learn more about this amazing mineral.

5. Chia has the trace mineral boron. You don't hear much about boron, but it, along with magnesium, helps the body put calcium to good use in bones and teeth. You can learn about trace minerals—the small nutrients that make a big difference in health—in this book.

6. Chia has omega-3 oil. That's the same kind of healthy oil in some types of fish. Health advisors usually encourage

eating fish for this type of oil but it's right there in the chia seed, without fishy flavor or fear of pollutants.

7. Chia has antioxidants. Antioxidants help fight free-radical damage. Free radicals exist in some unhealthy foods, in the natural environment, and in pollution of air, water, or food. They can cause signs of premature aging, inflammation, and more. Antioxidants in foods help neutralize these free radicals. They're also why chia has such an exceptional shelf life—did you know it will keep in a cool, dry place for two years? You can't do that with other nuts or seeds; their oil will go rancid. It's the high antioxidant content that keeps chia's omega-3 oil fresh.

8. Chia has B vitamins. By volume, one ounce of chia contains 2 percent vitamin B2 (riboflavin), 13 percent niacin, 29 percent thiamin, and trace amounts of all B vitamins. The various types of vitamin B are essential for you because they help your body get energy from foods. To process protein, for example, you'll need some B. For example, "according to the American Cancer Society, vitamins B1 and B2 assist in muscle and nerve development as well as heart function. Vitamin B3 assists in food digestion. Vitamins B5 and B12 aid in human growth and development. Vitamins B6 and B9 help increase your immunity to diseases and help create red blood cells. Vitamin B7 helps create hormones from the carbs and proteins you eat."[4]

All of these beneficial elements are packed into every tiny seed because nature is amazing! It's thought that the chia seed and its vigorous, fast-growing sprout are so nutrient-dense because of the harsh conditions the plant grows in. It must have enough nutrients

---

4 American Cancer Society, "B Vitamin Complex," http://www.cancer.org/treatment/treatmentsandsideeffects/complementaryandalternativemedicine/herbsvitaminsandminerals/vitamin-b-complex (Accessed 22 October 2013)

to take hold quickly, rise up fast, and begin photosynthesis in the sun, or face being blown away, pelted by sand, or starved out in the high altitude.

Does the Chia Plant Have Any Benefits?

Yes! The main feature of the chia plant is the special oil in the stems and leaves. Insects and other pests can't stand this oil. Because the plant really does take care of itself, you don't need pesticides to grow it. This helps make chia a really safe crop, especially if you're interested in close-to-nature, organic types of foods.

The second benefit is its preference for inhospitable areas. Because most chia is grown in areas where you couldn't raise other crops, the land hasn't been polluted with chemical fertilizers or runoff from previous crops.

The third benefit is that you can eat the sprouts. It's easy to sprout chia in your home. It will sprout almost anywhere, given a little bit of soil and water. The plant won't rise above the sprout stage unless the environmental conditions are correct though. When the sprout is about one to three inches high, you can clip it and eat it. The sprouts are very nutritious, but they have a distinct, spicy flavor. They can be added to salads or put on a burger. You can't eat a regular chia plant, though—only the sprout.

Is There Anything to Be Cautious Of?

When buying chia, be sure to look for seeds that were grown in an environment fairly close to the original dry, higher-altitude climate. Chia can, and should, be grown all over the world if that area has an appropriate climate.

If the chia plant doesn't dry up at the end of its season, it won't release the seeds from the center of its flowers. If it won't release the seeds, people will use chemical drying agents on the plants. This isn't regarded as a healthy practice. When you're looking for chia, be sure to select seeds with a normal market price. Some seeds that are very inexpensive won't have had the necessary screen filtering done for them. You may find weed seeds, tiny leaf bits, sticks, or even small stones mixed into the chia. These aren't harmful, but they are not attractive.

Chia Seed Color Differences

When looking at chia, you may see two colors of seeds. Chia is always patterned with little speckles or wavy lines, but the seeds come in two basic colors. The plants that make each color look about the same. Both have flowers and yield tiny, healthy seeds. But what you may not know is that the different colors of seeds have different nutritional values. Chia plants with purple flowers will yield brown seeds. These are called black chia, though each seed is a variety of different colors of brown, mottled together in a unique pattern. Plants with white flowers will produce only white seeds. These are a marbled mixture of white, gray, and yellow.

SO, WHAT'S THE DIFFERENCE?

The seeds are actually pretty similar in nutritional content, but if you want the best of both worlds, you need a brand of chia seed that mixes together both colors. There may be outrageous claims or bias around the Internet for one type of seed over the other. Some people prefer white chia for the cosmetic look of it in baked goods, (it doesn't make little black speckles in pale cakes or cookies). The best way to meet your diet and nutrition goals is to look at the facts for yourself. Some chia retailers sell only one type (color) of seed or meal, so be sure to get the facts first before you buy. Because if you get the right type of chia, you'll be getting all this, and more!

- Magnesium: fifteen times more than broccoli
- Calcium: six times more than whole milk
- Omega-3: nearly nine times the amount found in salmon
- Fiber: more than flaxseed and two times more than bran flakes
- Iron: nearly three times more than spinach
- Protein: chia has more than soy (chia has 2 grams of protein for every 10 grams of seeds, while tofu products generally have 1 gram per every 10 grams of product)

Now, take a look at the following nutrition rundown:

- Black seed protein: 4.7 grams per ounce
- White seed protein: 4.6 grams per ounce
- Black seed fiber: 10 grams per ounce
- White seed fiber: 10.8 grams per ounce
- Black seed cholesterol: 0 grams
- White seed cholesterol: 0 grams

Black seeds have more anthocyanins than white seeds. Anthocyanins are the pigments in fruits, vegetables, and seeds that give them a dark color. These pigments work as antioxidants, helping prevent free-radical damage. Examples of foods with lots of anthocyanins are dark plums, blueberries, and pomegranates. The darker-colored chia seeds, of course, will have more antioxidants than the white ones. The exact nutritional content of chia seeds can vary as well, depending on where they were grown. The climate for the growing year also influences the amount of omega-3 oils and protein the seeds have.[5]

---

5   ISO 9000 Certified Lab, "Chart Averages" http://www.azchia.com/black-chia-seeds-vs-white-chia-seeds/

You can learn more about the benefits of antioxidants later on in this book.

WHAT CAN YOU DO WITH CHIA?

There are almost as many ways to use chia as there are foods and drinks to think of! You can bake with chia, stir it into drinks, sprinkle it over sandwiches, blend it into smoothies, use it to thicken dressings, help blend flavors together in sauces, freeze it into popsicles, mix it into soups, and cook it in burgers. The possibilities are endless and so much fun. We'll explain each one and give great recipe examples too, to help you get started. Chia is so easy to use and so healthy that you'll want to use it every day. There are two basic forms of chia seeds. You can sprinkle dry seeds onto or into foods or drinks, or you can create chia gel with its own versatile set of uses.

What Is Chia Gel?

Chia has different applications whether it's wet or dry. Dry seeds can be sprinkled onto or stirred into almost anything. Wet seeds create chia gel. You'll see chia gel throughout this book, so it's important to understand how to make it (it's so easy) and how it can benefit you.

The chia seed really stands out among other types of seeds!

No other seed possesses such hydrophilic properties (i.e., being attracted to water). The microfibers on the outer coating of the seed allow it to absorb *nine* times its own weight in water. This is extremely beneficial for anyone who eats the seed, for a number of reasons.

But how does it work?

See the diagram below for a closer look at a chia seed. The seed in this image is many, many times larger than a real chia seed.

Chia will gel in anything that's not too acidic. You can make chia gel with grape juice but not grapefruit or lemon juice. For maximum versatility, you can gel it in filtered water, then add the gel to other drinks for foods whenever you like.

So, how do you make chia gel?

It's so easy that anyone can do it. For plain chia gel that can be used in almost anything, you can use this simple recipe:

CHIA GEL RECIPE

INGREDIENTS
1 tablespoon dry chia seeds
9 tablespoons filtered water (or other liquid)
A resealable container, such as a cup with a lid

INSTRUCTIONS
Stir together the chia seeds and water with a fork or shake a closed container to prevent clumping. Leave the mixture alone for ten to fifteen minutes on the countertop. When you return, you'll find that your container is now full of chia gel. It won't pour like water and it will have an altogether-new texture. You're now ready to use the gel in baking or any other food-related application. It's a great value too because every single tablespoon of chia seeds makes nine tablespoons of useful gel. Chia gel will keep for about one week in the refrigerator in a covered container.

There are plenty of specific uses for and benefits of chia gel. These include helping with weight loss, aiding digestion, promoting positive intestinal flora, and helping reduce toxins.

There are a few basic water-retaining benefits of the chia seed for you to be aware of (other benefits are covered later in the book):

Keeps the entire digestive process hydrated: Because the water absorbed by the seed is somewhat difficult to remove, it takes the digestive process a while to break down the soluble fiber and absorb the water. This means that as the seeds pass through the colon, they are slowly irrigating it on the way through. Keeping food moist is an important way to prevent maladies such as constipation and diverticulitis. The soluble and insoluble fibers act as a "sweeper" to keep food moving easily.

Provides calorie replacement: Because chia seeds have no flavor of their own, they distribute and take on the taste of whatever food or drink you add them to. If you want them to taste like grape juice, just mix them in. They'll hydrate with the grape juice and taste just like it. It's the same with any beverage of your choice, including tea.

Because of the dramatic increase in size of the hydrated seeds, when you eat them, you feel full. However, you are replacing calories from food you'd normally eat with zero-calorie water or other low-calorie drinks! For example, if you mix one tablespoon of chia seeds with nine tablespoons of water, you end up with nine tablespoons of filling, nutritious chia gel. This can then be used to displace the volume of foods, without altering their taste. The seeds themselves have calories, of course, due to their omega-3 oils, and protein. However, when you make chia gel, the bulk of the gel is water (or your beverage of choice) and fiber. Because fiber cannot be digested or broken down by the body, you cannot absorb any calories from soluble or insoluble fiber. For example, if you have one tablespoon of dry chia seeds, it has sixty-eight make chia gel, and you eat one tablespoon of chia gel, it has only 7.7 calories.

Cuts fat in baking: Chia gel can be used to substitute for up to half the butter or oil in baked recipes without altering the taste, texture, or baking method.

Makes for easier digestion: The liquid clings to the seed and is removed slowly throughout the digestive process. This keeps the colon hydrated, so that it's easy to move food through it. Insoluble fiber is found in the seed's outer coating. It's this type of fiber that isn't digested by the body and is sometimes called "roughage." It acts like a "sweeper," moving things along in the intestinal tract and preventing constipation.

Fiber isn't the only thing—remember the above points? Chia seeds have you covered on all of them. You can even literally see the viscous (i.e., appearing like a gelatin or gummy) fibers on the outside when you make chia gel. These help lower blood cholesterol and normalize blood glucose and insulin levels.

The most unique aspect of chia use in foods has to be the amazing ability to substitute for butter or oil in baked recipes. The idea of using seeds to replace up to half the fat in a recipe and then having the food still taste, cook, and look exactly the

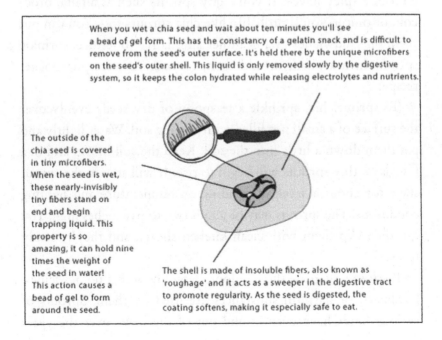

When you wet a chia seed and wait about ten minutes you'll see a bead of gel form. This has the consistancy of a gelatin snack and is difficult to remove from the seed's outer surface. It's held there by the unique microfibers on the seed's outer shell. This liquid is only removed slowly by the digestive system, so it keeps the colon hydrated while releasing electrolytes and nutrients.

The outside of the chia seed is covered in tiny microfibers. When the seed is wet, these nearly-invisibly tiny fibers stand on end and begin trapping liquid. This property is so amazing, it can hold nine times the weight of the seed in water! This action causes a bead of gel to form around the seed.

The shell is made of insoluble fibers, also known as 'roughage' and it acts as a sweeper in the digestive tract to promote regularity. As the seed is digested, the coating softens, making it especially safe to eat.

same, seems to be an outrageous claim. Indeed, no other seed in the world can live up to it, and that's because chia has that unique gelling property.

Sprouting Chia

Almost anyone can sprout chia seeds in his or her own home. Chia is a very vigorous plant that sprouts quite easily. That's why you can find it as a novelty gift item—it will even sprout on a textured clay surface. If you give chia seeds a little bit of dirt and a sunny windowsill, they'll sprout quickly. If the temperature and soil aren't correct (as in a low-altitude, desert-type sandy soil with dry air), the chia sprouts won't turn into chia plants.

Why would you want to sprout chia?

You can eat the sprouts! Chia sprouts, unlike the seeds, have a bit of a spicy flavor. If you enjoy sprouts such as alfalfa, broccoli, or onion, you'll probably like chia sprouts too. You can put them on sandwiches as a healthier alternative to lettuce, sprinkle sprouts into a salad, or add them to your favorite pita-pocket recipe.

To sprout chia, sprinkle a teaspoon of dry seeds evenly over the surface of a small pot filled with potting soil. Water lightly and pat them down a little into the soil. Keep the soil moist, and in a few days, tiny sprouts will begin to rise. It will stay in the sprout stage for about a week, depending on temperature and lighting conditions. The sprouts may be about two to five inches high. You can then clip them with clean kitchen shears, and they're ready to use.

Because you grow them indoors, you know that no pesticides, fertilizers, or harmful substances are used on them. Sprouts of various kinds have been in and out of the news over the years with regard to the possibilities of their contamination with *E. coli*. When you grow at home, you can see the safety of your food from start to finish. Because chia grows so quickly, it's a fun project for kids to do too.

Once you raise some sprouts, you can begin using them in your salads or wraps. Here's a recipe to get you started with your chia sprouts right away.

CHIA VEGGIE CRUNCH WRAPS

Chia sprouts add spiciness and a crunch factor to any salad or sandwich. Open your fridge and see what you have to work with and mix and match to your liking. This creamy avocado dressing will bind all your crunchy veggies and deli or leftover meats together in a terrific wrap to go. Just wrap in a wax paper packet, and a healthy lunch is at your fingertips, even on a busy day. This is another great way to enjoy chia!

INGREDIENTS:
DRESSING:
   ½ an avocado
   ⅓ cup low-fat sour cream
   1 tablespoon chia gel
   ½ teaspoon cumin

SUGGESTIONS FOR WRAP INGREDIENTS:
   Your wrap of choice (spinach wrap shown here)
   Chia sprouts
   Spinach or other dark greens
   Cucumber
   Tomato
   Onion

SUGGESTIONS FOR WRAP INGREDIENTS (CONT.):

Green apple
Carrot sticks, thinly sliced
Celery
Zucchini
Sweet peppers, thinly sliced
Radishes
Mushrooms
Pre-cooked cold asparagus
Deli ham, chicken, or beef, thinly cut
Chunk salmon
Low-fat cheese, thinly cut

INSTRUCTIONS:

Your options include any of the above healthy, tasty ingredients. You can mix and match to see what creates your favorite wrap. You can simply use what you've got in the fridge. Cut veggies such as cucumbers, tomatoes, zucchini, or bell peppers into long, thin slices. For a carrot, consider using a potato peeler to make thin, wide shreds that add crunch but aren't too thick.

For the dressing: In a small bowl mash the avocado with a fork or spoon. Stir in the sour cream, chia gel and cumin. Stir until thoroughly blended.

Warm the wrap in the microwave for a few seconds (if it has been refrigerated) so that it is pliable and will not crack when rolled and folded. On one half of the wrap, add a layer of your greenery, your protein, and your veggies of choice. Now, spoon the creamy avocado dressing over the mix and top it with your newly harvested sprouts. Fold over the other half of the wrap and roll tightly. For easy, non-messy enjoyment, roll the wrap into a sheet of wax paper, fold the ends in, then cut the roll in half.

Chia For Pets

Can you give chia seeds to your pets? Sure! Chia is healthy for pets too. Omega-3 oils are good for hair, skin, and nails. Many people have reported better fingernail health for themselves too when they use chia. Shiny fur and healthy skin need omega-3 oil. Pets' bones require calcium, just like yours do. Older pets at risk of arthritis are good candidates for chia as well, because omega-3 oil, calcium, and magnesium are all helpful in working against arthritis.

Chia for dogs: If you mix chia seeds into something your dog already likes, he or she won't even notice the tiny seeds. Wet dog food is ideal for this. Dogs may also just randomly eat chia seeds if you leave your chia lying around. It is thought that they can smell the oils in the seeds and some dogs think this is really tasty. Even though you can't smell the oil (most people think chia has no real scent at all), dogs can.

Chia for cats: Cats are complete carnivores. They won't just randomly eat seeds so you have to disguise them by adding a little bit to wet cat food.

Chia for birds: Chia is great for your seed-eating birds. It's easier for them to digest than flaxseeds, and most bird stores and bird-related retailers claim that the vitamins in chia help with feathering. Boron (a trace mineral in chia) also helps birds add calcium to their bones. The plant source calcium in chia is also easy to digest.

Chia for horses: Most horses really love the minimal flavor of chia. You can mix it into their normal feed. Some people who have tried giving chia to their horses report that the horses feel calmer when their diet includes chia. It could be the omega-3 oil. Omega-3s have been found to help promote brain health in humans, so they could do the same for horses.

A benefit that's just for horses: Soluble fiber can help clear sand from their digestive systems. Chia has soluble fiber that you can see, so it's effective for helping with sand clearing. Chia is high in soluble fiber, providing 27.6 grams of fiber for every 100 grams of seed. While an average human might take one tablespoon of chia per day or a dog could take one teaspoon, a horse is much larger and needs more. It can become expensive to give chia to horses if you're getting the premium, triple-screen-filtered, human food-grade chia. Instead, you can look for "animal grade" chia. What's the difference? Animal grade chia is still just as healthy, but it may not have had all of the filtering processes done for it. For instance, you might see a tiny leaf bit, a flower stamen, a weed seed, a petal, or some other tiny bit of material that would be objectionable in your baked goods but can easily be overlooked by a grazing animal. Because it is less filtered, you'll find that it is less expensive and can be easily bought in bulk quantities.

What if my pet gets into my chia seeds and eats a lot?

Pets don't always behave 100 percent of the time, and this can include eating too much or eating things they shouldn't. If your pets get into your seeds, make sure they have plenty of water available. For humans, if you eat a lot of fiber suddenly, you can get stomach cramps, as the fiber absorbs all the liquid that was present in the stomach all at once. Animals are the same way; they can get stomach cramps from too much fiber added too suddenly.

The other side effect of eating too much chia at once (and it's the same for humans as it is for pets of any kind) is loose stool as the body dismisses the extra fiber. Once all the chia is passed out of the system, the effect will stop.

Grinding Chia: Milled Chia and Chia Flour

Have you heard of ground chia? Sometimes you can see milled, or preground, chia for sale. Some people prefer the texture of ground chia over whole seeds. Ground chia will still gel (though not as much as whole seeds) and it still has no flavor of its own.

When buying ground chia, you'll want to look for "cold-milled" chia seeds. It's important that the chia isn't heated in the process of grinding. If it is, the healthy oils can come out onto the grinding equipment and then you won't benefit from them. Ideally, each seed should be cut into four pieces by tiny, specialized blades.

If you don't want to buy ground chia (it is always more costly than whole seed because of processing), you can grind chia yourself using a coffee grinder, a high-speed blender, or a food processor with a high-speed blade. It won't be as fine as industrially ground chia but it still works well enough.

Why would you want ground chia? There are a few reasons:

- You can change the texture of food with it.
- You can thicken smoothies or add texture to home-baked breads or muffins. Some people prefer the texture of ground chia in their food and it's easy to give it a try.
- If you have a digestive problem that lowers your ability to digest food regularly, ground chia could be a good choice for you. When the seed's shell is pre-broken, the body has an easier time accessing the nutrients. Issues such as having a part of the intestine removed, low stomach acid diagnosis, irritable bowel syndrome (where food can move too quickly through the intestine and fewer nutrients get absorbed), or diverticulitis are all good reasons to try ground chia.

Chia flour is less common than oat flour, rice flour, or potato flour. It's gluten-free but it has a "heavier" texture than regular white flour or whole wheat flour. If you're gluten intolerant, chia flour can be a baking option for you.

Baking with Chia

How would you like to be able to cut out half the fat from your favorite recipes? And what if you could do it without altering the taste or baking method?

It would be a cook's dream! And, now, this solution is finally within your grasp. One simple ingredient can cut half the butter, oil, and shortening from your recipes. Chia gel! For the recipe, see page 11.

Chia gel is as easy to use as butter or oil. It will keep for one week in a covered container in the refrigerator. (If you don't cover it, it will dry up.) Simply scoop the gel with a tablespoon measure and add it to your recipes just as you would butter.

Why does it work so well? Chia seeds don't have any flavor of their own. Instead, they take on the taste of whatever you add them to, and distribute that flavor. In that way, they can actually amplify flavors, and make your cooking even *more* delicious! But, be sure to use filtered water when you hydrate the seeds or any unsavory flavors in your tap water will be magnified. The healthy omega-3 oils and soluble fiber gelling action go to work moistening and enhancing the tastes in your recipe.

For example, if Grandma's favorite chocolate chip cookies recipe calls for eight tablespoons of butter, use four tablespoons of butter and four tablespoons of chia gel. Bake the cookies just as you normally would.

Are there any side effects? No, there are only side benefits! The exterior of the chia seed holds on to moisture, ensuring that your baked goods don't dry out while cooking and that they stay moist and rich-tasting for longer. These seeds also have high levels of antioxidants. Antioxidants are more than good for your body; they're nature's healthy preservative. They are what allows the seed to be dry-stored safely for more than two years without ever going rancid or decreasing in effectiveness. Don't try that with flax or millet; they'll go rancid as the oils inside spoil! It's these same anti-oxidants that keep food baked with chia fresh for longer periods.

Can you use chia gel as an egg substitute? In most cases, yes. However, if you take out the egg, you probably shouldn't also take out the butter or oil. Chia can generally be used to successfully replace either the egg *or* the butter in a recipe. The viscous nature of chia gel helps keep the texture of your egg-less baked item normal. Of course, you can't use it to substitute for something that rises on egg whites or relies on whipped egg whites for texture or lightness.

> To replace one regular size egg, use two tablespoons of chia gel.
>
> To replace butter or oil, use one tablespoon of chia gel per tablespoon of butter or oil removed from the recipe. You can generally replace up to half of the butter, oil, or shortening with gel and still keep the same texture and flavor of your food.

You can't whip chia gel and it doesn't help anything rise.

There are some great baked chia recipes in this book but if you'd like to try replacing butter or oil with chia gel in your own favorite recipes, that's a great idea too! You won't have to alter the baking time by much; generally, only a minute or two more of baking time should be added.

Most people don't realize how oily mainstream or prepared baked goods are. Just look at this comparison photo of a refriger-ated store-bought dough brand and the same type of cookie baked from scratch from the recipe on this page with chia in it:

The cookie on the left is the cookie made using the recipe from this book. The cookie on the right is a store-bought dough cookie. Look at what happens when you set each cookie on a piece of colored paper and wait ten minutes. The oil spots are *much* smaller on the chia side. This illustrates how much less fat you can use

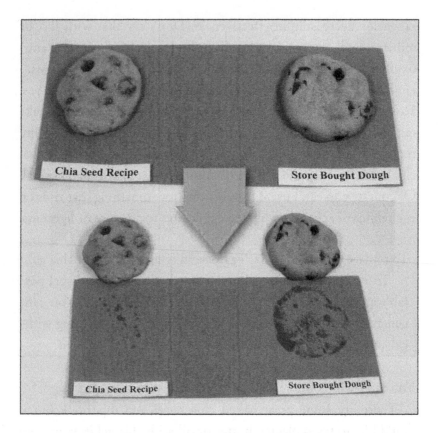

while baking a tasty cookie that looks and tastes just the same. You'll be amazed!

Would you like to make this cookie?

Here's the recipe so that you can see the results for yourself when you bake this chia treat.

CHEWY CHIA CHOCOLATE CHIP COOKIES

Chocolate chip cookies come in two basic textures: chewy and crispy. This recipe is for the chewiest, most melt-in-your-mouth-delicious chocolate chippers you'll have ever eat.

If you like crispy cookies, stay far away because these bake up puffy, light, and never oily. The soft, moist cookies are full of big, gooey chocolate chips. They taste fantastic hot from the oven and keep well in sealed containers. However, because they are moist and rich-tasting with no preservatives, they should be refrigerated after a few days to prevent mold. (Much like a bakery-fresh moist bread, these cookies need care to not go stale.)

Extra fact: Most cookie recipes make cookies of only *one* size. If you attempt to make the cookies at a size that is not described in the original recipe, you'll run into problems such as undercooking while edges burn or overdone cookies despite the baking time. These cookies can easily be made in any of *three* sizes!

- From ¼ cup scoops of dough at once for giant cookies to . . .
- 1 ½ tablespoon scoops for medium cookies, and . . .
- 1 ½ teaspoon scoops for small cookies

With this recipe, the size is totally up to you! Just adjust the baking time accordingly (see details in the recipe below). A big chocolate chip cookie can make a nice thank-you gift for someone you know. When it's homemade, it really shows you care, and you only need to spend minutes making them!

How could a chocolate chip cookie get even better?

What if it had *half* the fat of an ordinary cookie?

What if it tasted richer and chewier than an ordinary cookie?

And what if it had fiber and healthy nutrients as well?

The seemingly impossible becomes possible with this fantastic chocolate chip cookie recipe. In one easy batch, these could become your new favorites. Chia gel is your secret to a better-tasting, lower-fat cookie that has extra nutrition.

ULTRA CHEWY CHIA CHOCOLATE CHIP COOKIES

INGREDIENTS:

DRY INGREDIENTS:
  2 cups flour
  ½ heaping teaspoon baking soda
  ½ teaspoon salt
  ¼ cup white sugar
  1 cup brown sugar
  2 cups semisweet chocolate chips

WET INGREDIENTS:
  8 tablespoons butter (best if melted first)
  4 tablespoons chia gel
  ¼ cup applesauce (unsweetened)
  1 teaspoon vanilla
  1 whole egg
  1 egg yolk

INSTRUCTIONS:
First, preheat the oven to 325 degrees Fahrenheit and grease your cookie sheets. Mix the melted butter and both sugars until well blended. Then add the vanilla, applesauce, whole egg, and egg yolk. Stir again until thoroughly combined. Last, add in your chia gel and stir again. In another bowl, combine the rest of the dry ingredients (flour, baking soda, and salt) except the chocolate chips. Once the dry ingredients are mixed, add them slowly to the wet ingredients with a wooden spoon. Stir until just combined. Last, add in the two cups chocolate chips.

SUGGESTIONS:
If you're making large or medium cookies, you can use jumbo chocolate chips or chocolate chunks.

If you're making small cookies, regular chocolate chips work best.

Sizes:

If you use ¼ cup of batter per cookie, bake for about fifteen minutes (yields large cookies).

If you use 1 ½ tablespoons of batter per cookie, bake for about twelve minutes (yields medium cookies).

If you use 1 ½ teaspoons of batter per cookie, bake for about ten minutes (yields small cookies).

When done baking, the cookies will become golden brown. The edges may appear lightly toasted but the centers will still be soft and puffy. Be careful not to overbake.

This is just one example of using chia in baking. You can also use it in recipes that require shortening, vegetable oil, or margarine. It's not limited to cookies, by any means! You can make breads, muffins, cupcakes, cakes, tortes, pancakes, or waffles, all with half the fat. You can use the recipes in this book or use chia in your own favorites. More recipes are available at your fingertips on the Internet and in our other book, *The Chia Seed Cookbook*.

APPLE CHAI TEA CHIA MUFFINS

Chai tea is so comforting. The warm aroma of cinnamon, cardamom, and cloves wafting through your home just smells like relaxation. These muffins take a little bit of time to make but are a fabulous dessert or a breakfast treat for the weekend. Read the Sunday paper and enjoy!

Ingredients:
    2 chai tea bags
    1 cup boiling water
    ½ cup minced green apple
    2 eggs
    1 tablespoon vegetable oil
    2 tablespoons chia gel

¼ cup applesauce

⅔ cup brown sugar

2 teaspoons vanilla

¾ cup quick-cooking oatmeal (no sugar)

1 cup flour

1 teaspoon baking powder

½ teaspoon baking soda

1 teaspoon lemon zest

½ teaspoon cinnamon

Dash freshly cracked black pepper

INSTRUCTIONS:

Preheat your oven to 350 degrees Fahrenheit and apply cooking spray to or place cupcake wrappers in a muffin tin. Boil the cup of water and place the tea bags inside it to steep for about ten minutes. In a large bowl combine all the dry ingredients including the brown sugar. In a second bowl, beat the eggs with a fork until slightly fluffy. Combine the vegetable oil, chia gel, applesauce, vanilla, lemon zest, and black pepper with the egg mixture. Then stir in the chai tea (be sure to squeeze out all the tea goodness from the bags). Stir in the apple pieces. Pour the wet ingredient bowl into the dry ingredients. Stir until well blended. Depending on your muffin tin, this recipe makes about nine muffins. Bake for approximately twenty minutes or until an inserted toothpick comes out clean. Cool to room temperature on your baking rack before putting any uneaten muffins away in a sealed container.

OJ CRANBERRY BREAD

This rustic bread comes together quickly and smells so good while it is baking. It is a dense and moist bread with an explosion of flavors. You can serve this bread at breakfast or it complements a salad beautifully. OJ cranberry bread is just a little bit sweet and has no shortening, oil, *or* butter! Chia gel at work again!

Ingredients:

    1 cup all-purpose flour

    1 cup whole wheat flour

    ½ cup sugar

    2 teaspoons baking powder

    ½ teaspoon salt

    ½ teaspoon baking soda

    1 egg

    ½ cup orange juice, freshly squeezed (a naval orange works best in this application)

    3 tablespoons chia gel

    1 teaspoon orange zest

    1 cup coarsely chopped fresh or frozen (thawed) cranberries

Instructions:

Preheat your oven to 350 degrees Fahrenheit.

In a bowl combine the two types of flour, sugar, baking powder, salt, and baking soda. In a mini chopper, coarsely chop the cranberries. In a second bowl, whisk the egg and add the orange juice, zest, and chia gel. Add to the dry ingredients and stir until just incorporated. Fold in the cranberries.

Bake in a 5 × 3 inch loaf pan coated with cooking spray for approximately sixty minutes.

Let cool, then keep the bread wrapped to retain moisture.

Flavor Blending with Chia

Not only can chia enhance your baking, it can also help your other dishes taste better with its flavor-blending ability. It's that awesome soluble fiber gel again that works so well to help combine flavors in foods, drinks, and dressings. When you use chia, you may notice a smoother overall taste. You may also notice that some recipes say to wait before serving to let flavors blend. This is to help ensure that the chia seed fiber does its job for you.

You can use chia seeds in your favorite recipes for dressings, smoothies, sauces, soups, and so much more. Sprinkle in chia, stir it into sauces, or use gel premade with filtered water to start your flavor-blending action. Gel is best used when something is not very citrus heavy (i.e., acidic) or has vinegar as chia won't gel with vinegar or overly acidic items. To get a firsthand demonstration of how chia flavor blending works, try these recipes that highlight fresh, fantastic flavors!

CHIA MELON BERRY SPLASH!

This is a great green smoothie. Don't be afraid of the green color; you won't taste the greens at all. It's very fresh, melon-y, and energizing. If you have kids who hate eating greens, a tropical-themed smoothie could be a good way to present them. The banana and cantaloupe keep the smoothie tasting sweet, while the grated ginger aids in digestion and adds just a little zing.

INGREDIENTS:

½ cup milk of your choice (almond or rice milk is recommended)
2 handfuls of fresh spinach
1 cup hulled strawberries
1 banana
1 cup cantaloupe chunks
1 teaspoon grated ginger root
1 tablespoon dry chia seeds
1 lime, zested and juiced (or 2 tablespoons lime juice)

INSTRUCTIONS:

Place the milk and spinach in a blender. Blend to chop the leaves to a tiny, bite-size consistency. Add the remaining ingredients and blend. Let this stand in the fridge for about ten minutes, then you're ready to enjoy.

GREEN SALAD WITH CHUNKY CRANBERRY VINAIGRETTE

This is a "whatcha-got-in-the-house" veggie salad. The chunky cranberry vinaigrette adds a nutrient-dense zing to any veggie salad. You can mix and match the contents of your fridge to make this most excellent salad. We buy cranberry bags while they are in season and freeze them so that we may have them all year long— cranberries are not just for the winter holidays and sauces loaded with sugar.

INGREDIENTS:
FOR THE VINAIGRETTE:
   ¼ cup olive oil
   3 tablespoons red wine vinegar
   ⅓ cup fresh or frozen cranberries (thawed)
   1 tablespoon Dijon mustard
   3 teaspoons agave nectar or honey
   2 cloves of garlic, minced
   2 tablespoons chia gel
   Several grinds of black pepper

FOR THE SALAD BED:
   ½ cup dry brown rice (makes 1 cup when cooked)
   1 orange
   1 tablespoon of dry chia

SALAD MIX-INS:
   Cauliflower florets
   Bite-size green apple pieces
   Broccoli florets

Kiwi slices

Raspberries

Sunflower seeds (or other nuts of choice, for crunch)

INSTRUCTIONS:

HOW TO PREP THE SALAD:

Start by zesting and sectioning the orange while reserving the juice. Start cooking the brown rice per the directions on the package. Add a tablespoon of chia and the orange juice to the rice while it cooks. Simmer for the allotted time. Cool to room temperature and add the zest. Stir to combine.

If you choose to include shredded chicken to add more protein, you can use leftover chicken or a rotisserie chicken or grill a chicken breast (indoors or outdoors). Cool the chicken to room temperature before adding to the salad.

HOW TO MAKE THE CHUNKY DRESSING:

In a mini chopper or food processor (even your blender will work), add the cranberries and chop to just a very chunky consistency. You don't want to overchop at this point. Then, add all the other dressing ingredients and pulse just a little to combine. Let this stand in the fridge for about ten minutes to help the chia blend the flavors together.

HOW TO PLATE THE SALAD:

Lay a bed of orange-brown rice first. Place the greens, veggies, and fruit on top along with chicken if desired. This dressing is nice and chunky so it will cling to your ingredients for a blast of flavor with every bite. Dress with the cranberry vinaigrette and enjoy!

Note: We used mixed greens (heavy on the spinach), shredded mixed cabbage, orange sections (left over from the rice preparation), diced red onion, chopped green apple, broccoli and cauliflower florets, kiwi, a few leftover raspberries, and sunflower seeds. This is a "whatcha-got" recipe. Pear, celery, crumbled blue cheese, and nuts of choice all work really well here and are quite tasty.

CHIA SALMON PATTY WITH LIGHT LEMON SAUCE

We all hear that we should eat more fish to get our omega-3s, but fish farming and the unsanitary conditions often associated with this process, plus the issue of mercury in wild predatory fish, may leave you gritting your teeth. You can easily cancel out the health benefits of fish if it contains toxins such as mercury, antibiotics, or harmful chemicals and pollutants. Often we will opt for canned wild Alaskan salmon to make this patty. You'll find the taste light and freshened up with the lemon. Cross your fingers that you have an extra patty because it makes a great pita lunch with salad trimmings the following day. Makes four patties.

INGREDIENTS:

FOR THE PATTIES:
    1 15-oz can of Alaskan wild salmon
    1 egg
    1 tablespoon dry chia seeds
    1 garlic clove (minced)
    1 lemon (zested and juiced)
    1 ½ teaspoons Old Bay spice blend
    2 tablespoons bread crumbs
    A few stems of parsley (lightly chopped)

FOR THE SAUCE:
    ¼ cup low-fat sour cream
    1 teaspoon lemon juice and zest
    Dash cayenne pepper

INSTRUCTIONS:

Press out the liquid from the salmon and pick through it to remove the skin and bones. Place the salmon and the other patty ingredients in a bowl. Mix by hand to combine. Press into four patties and let the patties rest for about ten minutes so that the dry chia absorbs the extra moisture in the patties. Grill indoors or broil to make the patties crispy on the outside and cooked thoroughly, about three to four minutes per side.

To make the sauce: Mix all sauce ingredients together in a small bowl with a spoon. The easy sauce adds just the right amount of freshness to your patty.

Losing Weight with Chia

Chia is great as a general supplement for health but by using it in specific methods outlined in this section of the book, it makes a great, safe weight loss helper too. The gelling property can be used to fight hunger, while the fiber improves digestion and speeds food through the digestive tract.

Any dieter knows that hunger is a main enemy of trying to lose weight. When you're hungry, you're probably thinking about food. When you're hungry, you're more likely to have cravings for certain foods and also more likely to give in to them. When you're hungry, you're more likely to overeat at mealtimes. Wouldn't it be great to be able to stop hunger at will, whenever it happened? What if you could do it easily, safely, *and* cheaply? How do you think that would impact your weight loss efforts?

If you think this could make a huge difference not only in your success, but the *ease* of success, you can't miss out on these methods.

How do chia seeds keep you feeling full? When the chia seed is exposed to water or other liquids, it begins to hydrate. This means that the fibers on the outside of the seed (almost too small to see with the naked eye) begin to trap moisture and form it into a gel. Each seed forms its own big bead of gel that is not easily removed. When you eat this seed/gel combination, your body treats it like a big piece of food, not the zero-calorie water that it really is! The seeds themselves, of course, have calories, due to their omega-3 oils and protein. However, when you make chia gel, the bulk of the gel is water and fiber. Because fiber cannot be digested or broken down by the body, you cannot absorb any calories from soluble or insoluble fiber. The seeds are tiny and healthy, but it's their ability to absorb *nine times* their own weight in water that keeps you feeling full. This means that you can use even one teaspoon of seeds to get rid of hunger whenever you want. For example, one tablespoon of dry chia seeds has sixty eight calories, but one tablespoon of chia gel has only 7.7 calories.

CUT APPETITE BEFORE MEALTIME METHOD

Want to eat less at mealtimes? Add a tablespoon or two of chia gel to a glass of water and drink it about fifteen to twenty minutes before a meal. The stomach is notoriously slow in getting signals to the brain. The "oh, something is here, I might be a little bit full now" signal can take about fifteen minutes to reach the brain. If you're not starving at mealtime, you won't eat as much. You should experiment to find the amount of chia gel that's right for you.

SNACK REPLACEMENT METHOD

Some weight loss efforts can be sabotaged by snacking. If hunger compels you to visit the vending machine in the afternoon between lunch and dinner, you can substitute that snack with chia. Grabbing a glass of juice or a cup of tea with chia gel in it will help you feel full.

ADD CHIA TO YOUR FOOD

Adding dry chia to food by sprinkling it over a salad or using a chia dressing can help you feel full faster, with less food. You'll have to experiment with the amount of chia that's right for you. Chia also keeps you feeling full longer. If you are usually hungry by lunchtime, try adding chia to breakfast; you'll likely find that it's very easy to make it all the way to lunch without feeling hungry. Everyone will need a different amount to achieve the desired result, so feel free to experiment to get the quantity that's right for your goals.

HOW DO CHIA SEEDS HELP BALANCE BLOOD SUGAR AND PROVIDE YOU WITH MORE ENERGY?

Would you work out more if you *felt* like it?

What if you weren't too tired to do all sorts of fun activities that also burn calories? The chia seed can help with that. Chia is one of the few plant sources of complete protein. Usually, complete protein is found only in animal products. It provides you with healthy, steady energy. Blood sugar is also important in keeping you energized. It may spike after meals and leave you feeling rundown later. Ever feel like you need an afternoon nap for no real reason? Blood sugar is probably the culprit. Once again, it is the seed's fiber and gelling action to the rescue. The two kinds of fiber present in every seed (soluble and insoluble) slow down the body's conversion of carbohydrates into sugars. This results in blood sugar that's more even throughout the day and gives you the steady, never jittery or "crash-prone" energy you crave. Caffeine highs and sugary drinks will never provide that kind of long-lasting energy.

Good digestion is a part of weight loss. When your body is metabolizing food smoothly, easily, and with enough hydration, the toxins that might keep you rundown are flushed away. Insoluble fiber does not add calories because it cannot be digested by the body. Instead, it acts as roughage, keeping digested food moving along smoothly. The gel formed by the soluble fibers of the seeds keeps the colon hydrated.

Did you know that being deficient in minerals or vitamins can create a craving for food?

For instance, if you're low on calcium, you may want to eat lots of cheese and ice cream. Or you might want extra servings of pasta with cheesy or creamy sauce, driving up the calorie count with milk fats and starchy carbs. By balancing your vitamins and minerals with chia, you can curb cravings that might tempt you. By weight, chia has more calcium than whole milk. It also has magnesium and boron, essential trace minerals used in the absorption of calcium and other vitamins.

Can you eat a fat to lose fat? That's what *International Journal of Obesity* reported in a study of dieters.[6] In the study, people on the diet who were also supplementing with omega-3 oil, lost more weight than people who didn't use this healthy oil. Omega-3 oil, commonly found in fish such as salmon and cod liver oil, is a healthy oil your body needs for cellular health. It may even help raise good cholesterol, improve digestion, and relieve some types of arthritis pain.

But where did all the omega-3 go? Is its loss part of the obesity cause? Animal fats (real butter, cream, etc.) are seen to have saturated fats (long seen as the bad guy) and have been phased out in favor of plant-based oils such as corn, sunflower, and rapeseed. These plant oils may be unsaturated, and they may boast a long shelf life, but they also are loaded with omega-6, the less healthy of the oils. When you consume too much omega-6, it can cause

---

6   *International Journal of Obesity*, "Effect of Dietary Fish Oil on Body Fat Mass and Basal Fat Oxidation in Healthy Adults," *Nature*, http://www. nature.com/ijo/journal/v21/n8/pdf/0800451a.pdf (Accessed 22 October 2013)

inflammation that may lead up to a buildup of cholesterol in the arteries. Some omega-6 is needed for cellular health but too much of it can be a problem.

In all, chia helps you lose weight in six ways: it stops hunger, quiets cravings for food, improves digestion, gives you the energy to be active, balances blood sugar, and helps restore the omega-3 balance. If "big pharma" ever found a pill that could do all that, you can bet they'd charge an arm and a leg for it. But enough chia for one month is far less than $1 per day, all-natural, and has zero risk. When you want to lose weight, keep it off, and stay healthy and energized the whole time, nothing can beat the chia seed. You have nothing to lose but the excess weight, so see for yourself how great these seeds really are!

IS PROTEIN REALLY GOOD FOR WEIGHT LOSS?

Everyone's heard the standard weight loss advice, which is to eat less fat and eat more whole grains. But can eating *more* of something really help you lose weight too? Amidst all the whole grain and vegetable frenzy, an important key for health is being sadly neglected, and that is protein. Protein is the building block of muscle tissue, whether it's your legs, your heart, or your stomach—they're all muscle, and you need them all in top shape to stay healthy. Muscle tissue actually even burns fat while just sitting around! So the more muscle you have, the easier you'll find it to burn off fat.

If you wanted to build a brick wall, you wouldn't reach for cardboard, glass, or cloth. You would reach for bricks. It's the same way within your body. If you want to build muscle, you reach for protein, not fat, carbohydrates, or fiber. Make no mistake, fats, carbs, and fiber are all important for health as well, and everyone needs some of them, however, none of them will do the same job that protein will for you. You hear about protein for building muscle (whether in growing children, or maintaining healthy muscle mass in old age), but you seldom hear about using it for weight loss.

Protein is not stored like fat, or converted into fat by the body. Carbohydrates, sugars, fats, and oils can all be converted into (your) fat. Fat is a storehouse of energy that the body can choose to use at any time. It prevents starvation and provides a ready source of energy when others aren't available. However, protein is an immediate energy source that's very efficient. You'll hear about the supposed "fat-burning switch" in various protein drinks and powders. There may not be an actual button to press, but by eating plenty of quality protein, you are giving your body a signal that "the food supply is fine; you don't need to keep storing fat."

Is your protein of good quality? There are an abundance of "food items" masquerading as protein that aren't actually of good quality. These can include overcooked foods, foods treated with radiation (it doesn't change the look or the taste but it wrecks the nutrients while killing bacteria), foods with too many preservatives, and foods with too many chemicals used to grow or process them. For example, some chickens are fed arsenic (that's poisonous to humans and birds) to force them to gain weight. Of course, it's still present in the meat when you get it, lowering the nutritional value. Unhealthy animals of any kind won't have healthy meat. So, it's best to try to stay away from processed meats when trying to get your protein.

Choosing the right type of protein is important for quality. Picking up a bucket of fried chicken may provide protein but it is clearly not your best bet for health and maintaining a healthy weight. Choosing your protein is easy and healthy when you look at this list:

- *Eggs:* Eggs are a good source of protein, but free-range eggs are the best. Chickens who are outside in the sun add lots of important vitamin D to their eggs. Eggs from the healthiest and happiest chickens are a real powerhouse of nutrients and protein for you. Typical egg mills are a terrible place for hens, with poor living conditions and a bad diet. Their terrible circumstances lead them to make poor eggs.

- *Grass-fed beef:* Cows were meant to eat grass and be outdoors in the sun, moving around. A natural diet and proper exercise keeps most animals healthy without the need for excessive antibiotics, hormones, and medicines. *E. coli* (the terrible bacteria) is almost nonexistent in grass-fed cows. When animals are raised in natural conditions, they produce better, healthier meat. Eating antibiotics and hormones isn't good for you, but they're passed along to you when you eat most factory meats.

- *Fish and chicken:* Again, the wilder, the better. Wild-caught Alaskan salmon and outdoor chickens are the healthiest. Avoiding large fish such as swordfish, shark, and tuna will also limit your possible mercury exposure. Wild salmon and Norwegian cod provide healthy omega-3 oil and protein.

- *Beans and nuts:* Animals aren't the only source of healthy protein. Plant protein usually isn't complete, but by combining different kinds of protein in the same meal, you can still get all the amino acids you need. Combinations such as grains and legumes (e.g., wheat or rice, and beans), corn and beans, or seeds and beans will provide the essential amino acids. Protein can contain up to twenty amino acids. Your body can make all of them (via combining different nutrients from foods you eat) except for eight. The final eight you have to consume. Plant sources are also wonderful to consider as they don't have the added fat or expense of meats.

- *Chia seeds:* The chia seed is rare among plants in that it is a 100 percent complete protein. It does not have the plant estrogens that soy has. Usually, complete protein is found only in meat. With vegetable sources, you must combine different sources to get complete protein. However, with these seeds, you don't have to. They're 23 percent protein by weight too, which is a nice, high ratio for a plant. The seeds have no flavor, so you can add them to anything you already like to eat, from cereals, to salads, to sandwiches without altering the taste. It's so easy to use that there's no excuse not to reach for this easy protein boost!

How else does protein contribute to helping you lose weight? Protein does not raise blood sugar levels. When your insulin is regulated and balanced (not spiking with sugar or carb overload), your body won't want to store excess fat in case the quick-burning carbs suddenly run out.

When your body has plenty of protein each day, it is not in survival mode. It will be much more likely to allow any fat stores to be burned off because real, healthy fuel is always available. Remember, your body doesn't know that food is always, and will always, be readily available.

Give your body the "fat-fighting signal" by adding easy, healthy, and tasty protein to your diet!

WHAT CAN SABOTAGE YOUR WEIGHT-LOSS EFFORTS?

Let's take a moment to look at the top three most abused items that food chemists love to use. These would be sugar, fats, and salt. Food chemists love these big three because you can create actual food addictions by combining them in different ways. For example, did you know that a food with just the right balance of sugar and salt will tempt you to eat more of it? The body has natural "off switch" that it generally can use when you've had enough of something that is *either* sweet or salty. You can crave salty food, such as a bag of chips, but after eating a handful or two of them, you'll want a drink or the chips won't be so appealing any longer. (Crave-driven eating is not the same thing as "mindless eating," where someone eats long after they are full, or because of inattention to the food.)

Food chemists can combine sugars and salts so that the food never triggers the "I've had enough" signal in the brain (called sensory specific satiety in the food industry). There are real, highly paid food scientists out there with the sole goal of getting each consumer to eat more of the food the scientists were assigned to make even more addictive. There's so much money in the food and snack industry that millions of dollars every year are devoted to food chemistry and creating food addictions.

With a few quick, eye-opening facts about the big bad three, you can put this knowledge to work for you and your family. We will teach you how to train your brain and show you how using chia seeds in your diet and the new healthier lifestyle will enhance your energy level, your mood, and your sense of well-being. You can break away from these snack foods that were created specifically to be addictive. Once you up your nutrition levels and feel better each day, you will never want to go back to the way it was.

HIDDEN AND ADDED SUGARS

Well, we all know how bad sugar is for you and for maintaining a healthy body weight and good blood chemistry. The issue isn't with just plain sugar or the sugar in natural fruits, it's with the overuse of sugar in so many products today. Did you know *just how bad* too much sugar is for you?

The health problems we hear about in the news the most are obesity and diabetes. But are you ingesting hidden sugars? You know when you decide to have a sweet snack in the afternoon, a donut in the morning, a soft drink . . . you are consuming sugar. However, there could be danger lurking in your kitchen cupboards and in your fridge! Read the ingredient labels on BBQ sauces, salad dressings, low-fat snacks, peanut butter, all bread and bread products, little packages of instant oatmeal . . . the list goes on and on. Especially watch your low-fat items. Removing fats tends to also remove flavor. Most products will compensate by adding either lots of sugars or lots of salt.

Don't be fooled when you see these words: high fructose corn syrup, corn syrup, corn solids, beet sugar, fruit juice/concentrate, glucose, ethyl maltol, galactose, honey, maltose, molasses, rice syrup, dextrose, barley, malt, caramel, dextrose, treacle, golden syrup, maple syrup, sucrose, malt syrup, and cane juice. These are all types of sugar. They're in many more products than you would think. Do you think prepackaged microwave meatballs without sauce need sugar? Some companies do. Look for sugar in really strange places on prepackaged foods. Lots of things you'd never suspect have added sugar.

Nutritionists call sweet foods "anti-nutrients." This is because they replace whole, nutritious food choices and they actually consume nutrients while being digested. For instance, both a fresh peach and a donut have sugar. However, the peach has natural fruit sugars and a host of other nutrients, while the donut just has processed sugar and white flour without fiber. All foods require vitamins and minerals to provide the energy to be digested. (Remember the function of B vitamins!) When you consume "anti-nutrients," you make your body work harder, and you can even cause inflammation.

What can you do? Read the labels! Read the label of anything you buy before you eat it. Make sure that hidden sugar is not sabotaging your efforts at better health. Don't forget that food companies are in the business of making money, not watching what you eat. Making food at home is a great idea because you will always know what's going into that snack, meal, or dessert. You can also customize foods with the seasonings that you like best.

ARTIFICIAL SWEETENERS CAN SABOTAGE YOUR EFFORTS

Unless you are living under a rock and haven't been keeping up with the news, studies are showing that the use of artificial sweeteners (with zero calories) is just as unhealthful as the use of over-sugared products—and maybe even more so.

Why? These products, all many times sweeter than natural sugars in any form, can and do train your brain to want more sweet satisfaction. When you're used to the sweetness level of artificial sweeteners, natural sugars are never sweet enough for you. Your body needs glucose for cell respiration and a source of energy. If you are giving your body only sugar substitutes, it will never be satisfied. You'll crave more food and more artificial sweeteners and start the cycle again.

Some people also experience side effects from consuming artificial sweeteners. It can be something very mild and unnoticeable, such as added inflammation in the digestive tract. Or, in the case of aspartame, it can make some people much hungrier when they use it. Does added hunger ever help anyone's weight loss efforts?

For example, the *Journal of Toxicology and Environment* found evidence that aspartame, sucralose, and neotame can cause weight gain in people who try to use it to lose weight.

The journal also reveals that sucralose

- Reduces the amount of friendly bacteria in your intestines by 50 percent
- Increases the pH level in your intestines, and causes an acidic body chemistry
- Sugar substitutes may affect the way medicine is (or is not) absorbed in the body[7]

---

7   *Journal Toxicology* via Mercola.com, "New Study of Splenda (Sucralose) Reveals Shocking Information About Potential Harmful Effects," http://articles.mercola.com/sites/articles/archive/2009/02/10/new-study-of-splenda-reveals-shocking-information-about-potential-harmful-effects.aspx   (Accessed 22 October 2013)

The reduction of friendly bacteria will cause an imbalance of good versus bad bacteria in your digestive system, resulting in various digestive maladies which can include weight gain as the bad bacteria don't process fats properly.

What can you do? Read all labels, especially for flavored beverages. Currently, there are almost zero choices in the market for "easy to-go" flavorings (both liquids and powders that you add to water to make a beverage). Nearly every single one will contain sucralose or aspartame. Those "zero-calorie" sport, health, or diet beverages? It's often the same case with those.

You can opt for natural, sweeter-than-sugar sweeteners too. Look for products that use stevia (derived from a leaf—real stevia will have leaf particles), xylitol (derived from tree bark), or monk fruit extract (a liquid extracted from the lo han guo fruit of Asia). These natural sweeteners are many times sweeter than sugar and you can use them in your beverages instead of chemical sweeteners.

Of course, if you're diabetic and can't eat that much of Mother Nature's sugars and you need a sugar "fix," well, we say, stick with the less harmful sugar substitutes such as stevia or xylitol.

SPICE UP YOUR LIFE!

Food has to taste good. Food chemists would have you believe that you *need* the big three (sugar, fats, and salts) to have food that tastes good. It's just not true because herbs and spices add great flavor *and* great nutritional power to food. No one would want to stick to healthier eating habits if all food was gross, bland, or boring. You have to want to choose the healthier food options, and there's no other way to do that than through great taste. While food chemists fiddle around trying to remove one of the big three to make something "healthier," they end up adding more of the other two members of the big three and then the food isn't as healthy anymore.

You don't often see packaged and highly processed foods relying on spices for flavoring. Keep in mind that with food manufacturers, the bottom line is number one. If they can choose a spice substitute, something that tastes similar, or just plain old salt, they generally do. This isn't a problem for you when you make food at home. You can choose the amount of seasonings and those you like best. Because you're not an industrial manufacturer, you can spend just pennies seasoning your favorite foods with simple, store-bought choices or herbs from the local farmer's market.

All of the herbs and spices people use in cooking add so much flavor to a meal and all cultures have their favorites. But did you know how beneficial adding a variety of spices can be? Increasing your use of spices or trying new herbs and spices will add more and different nutrients to your meal plans. Just look at all the health benefits each of these common herbs and spices adds to your meals beside great flavors:

- *Cinnamon:* provides magnesium, iron, and calcium, is a proven anti-inflammatory and helps control and regulate blood sugar
- *Basil:* provides vitamins A and K, calcium, iron, potassium, flavonoids (which sharpen your recall), and eugenol (which protects you from harmful bacteria)
- *Garlic:* provides magnesium, vitamins B6, B1, and C, tryptophan, selenium, and phosphorus; also lowers blood cholesterol levels and blood pressure, is anti-inflammatory, is an antioxidant, and is an antibacterial/antiviral agent
- *Ginger:* provides magnesium, potassium, copper, and vitamin B6; can help with stomach upsets and is an anti-inflammatory agent
- *Chili powder and paprika:* provides vitamins A and C, potassium, and iron; capsicum in all peppers fights inflammation,

improves circulation, lowers cholesterol, and boosts the immunity system

- *Parsley:* provides vitamins A, K, and C and is a good source of folate and iron; is also a great antioxidant and neutralizes carcinogens
- *Oregano:* provides vitamins K, A, and C, magnesium, iron, and omega-3s; is also an antioxidant and has antibacterial properties
- *Onions:* provide vitamins C and B6, manganese, folate, tryptophan, and chromium; improve cardiovascular health, are anti-inflammatory, and are antibacterial agents
- *Thyme:* provides vitamin K, iron, and magnesium; is antimicrobial and an antioxidant
- *Cardamom:* provides magnesium, iron, zinc, and potassium; detoxifies the body's kidneys and bladder and detoxifies the body overall
- *Cloves:* contain eugenol, which is found to naturally protect the body from environment pollutants, and is a known anti-inflammatory agent; clove oils can be a mild anesthetic and an antibacterial agent as well
- *Rosemary and sage:* are high in carnosol, a cancer-fighting agent and phenolic acid; also are memory and mood enhancers and anti-inflammatory agents
- *Curry powder:* includes curcumin, and turmeric, which is shown to prevent some cancers, and vitamin C, and is shown to promote cognitive abilities as well as bad cholesterol reduction (curry powders are different for every region, but all contain some turmeric and curcumin).[8]
- *Tarragon:* has antioxidant properties to neutralize free radicals and aids in digestion

---

8   John La Puma MD and Rebecca Powell Marx, *Chef MD's Big Book Of Culinary Medicine*, (Crown Publishing 2008), 14 and 75

- *Mustard:* is rich in selenium and magnesium, which have phytonutrient compounds that inhibit and prevent gastro-intestinal cancer and have been shown to reduce migraine attack
- *Cumin:* may aid in digestion and helps control hypoglycemia
- *Ground peppercorns:* contain piperidine, piperetin, and piperine chavicine compounds which encourage the production of acid in the stomach to digest foods; has antibacterial properties and helps the body absorb vitamins and minerals

This is just a short list of the most common herbs and spices! There are many others waiting at the spice shelf for you to discover. Now that you know how good each of these seasonings is for you, see how many of them you can find in recipes in this book. The MySeeds Chia Test Kitchen is never shy about flavor.

NUTRITION VERSUS CALORIES

If you are trying to lose weight, counting calories may not be the way to go. The choices you make when you go to the grocery store and the way you prepare foods have a huge impact on your health, your sense of well-being, and your weight. The modern diet that includes packaged foods, overprocessed foods, and gimmicky snacks often tries to hide calories. Unhealthy calories include saturated fats, white flour that contributes nothing to your nutrition, and overcooked foods that have lost their nutrients in exchange for a lengthy shelf life. Calorie counting and label reading—it may be buyer beware.

What about the calories per serving? If you're counting calories, you're probably reading labels. That's a great first step to knowing just what's in your food. However, you can't always trust the label. Many people think the calorie count is how many calories are in the package. Lots of foods have a serving size that's much smaller than you would think. For instance, a bottled drink may seem like one serving, but if you read the label, it could be two or three servings. Most people will drink a whole bottled beverage in a sitting. The calories listed are always per serving, so you would need to check the serving size as well.

Also, "Legally, food companies can be up to 20 percent off on the calorie count,"[9] says Dr. Darya Pino, PhD, Food Scientist. You can guess which side of the 20 percent off they err on. If it will make a product look better and tempt more people to buy it, they will definitely want to err on as much of the low side as they can.

Always check the serving size before you eat. Also, if you're trying to lose weight, assume the food has more calories than advertised. (And if you're plateauing, this may be part of the reason why.)

Your body needs calories, yes, to provide energy and to keep you alive. The calories included in macronutrients are carbohydrates, proteins, and fats. These macronutrients are so heavily consumed in the standard American diet that in 2009 more than 50 percent of people in America were considered obese. Let's not fight. Tackle this the smart, the easy, and the healthy way. You can't sprinkle chia seeds on a sugary and fat-laden donut and say, "Now I'll be healthier and lose weight," but with more knowledge and chia on your side, you can start training yourself and your brain.

Almost everyone really needs more vital nutrients. Micronutrients need to be a part of your body's chemistry. These little helpers are the key to steady energy and will help you ward off diseases and colds as well as let your body find its natural weight and natural body rhythms.

---

9 Dr. Darya Pino, PhD, "Biggest Food Label Lies," Delish.com, http://www.delish.com/recipes/cooking-recipes/calories-per-serving-biggest-food-label-lies#slide-9 (Accessed 18 October 2013)

Every plant has a different ratio of carbs, proteins, and fats. Each plant also has a varied assortment of enzymes, vitamins, and micronutrients. Consuming a large variety of different plants such as fruits, veggies, loads of greens, nuts, and seeds such as chia will all provide the *best* nutrient dense calories for the best, healthiest you. If these foods are prepared properly, you can practically eat as much volume as you would care to!

The proteins in plants are very easily digested and used by the body. Protein does not necessarily mean a giant slab of cooked animal. Most people associate protein only with two sources: meat and dairy products, such as whey. However, greens, lentils, legumes, quinoa, and chia all have protein. It is important to have a little protein at each meal. A complete protein helps keep you full and evens out your blood sugar levels. Not many plant-based foods are a complete protein that includes the eight essential amino acids your body cannot manufacture. Go chia! These little seeds offer a complete protein.

Just in case you were absent at school that day: What are amino acids? They are the building blocks of protein. Your digestive system breaks down proteins into their types of amino acids. The body then rearranges these amino acids into new proteins that the body requires.

So, as some of our MySeed Test Kitchen members are fond of chanting, "We are not rabbits! We are not rabbits eating only salads!" We will offer many ideas of foods that are filling, tasty, and nutrient dense, not just another salad. We don't offer a calorie count on any of our recipes. If you know that the calories are from healthy foods and that you're getting plenty of fiber, you'll feel full without worrying about getting too many calories from hidden sources or unhealthy saturated fats.

A LITTLE WORD ABOUT FATS

Too many modern sources rush to blame fats of all kinds for the weight problems that many people are experiencing. They act as if eating a fat will turn it immediately into fat somewhere on your body. It just doesn't work that way. If you eat a steak, does some part of you change into a cow? No. Fats are the same way. There are three main fat sources in anyone's diet. There are vegetable fats (e.g., olive oil, coconut oil, or avocados), there are animal fats (found in various meats, as well as cheeses, milk, and butter), and then there are manufactured or altered fats that have had chemical processing for one reason or another.

Saturated fats are found in animal products. These were blamed for being very unhealthy for quite some time in the media.

Trans fats or partially hydrogenated fats are man-made fats created by forcing hydrogen into vegetable oils to make them more solid at room temperature. This also extends the shelf life of some foods. Both of these characteristics are good for the bottom line, but they may not be good for you.

Monounsaturated fats are found in some plants such as avocados, olive oil, and peanuts. These fats can lower your cholesterol and reduce inflammation, which keeps your blood vessels healthy. These fats include omega-3s.

The "good" fats are required by the body for managing the heart, reproduction, and fetal development, managing the health of your brain and eyes, and helping maintain normal inflammation. So we all need to get more omega-3s in our diet.

Essential fatty acids (EFAs) provide needed nutrition for most all body functions. The alphabet letters are as follows:

- *ALA* stands for alpha-linolenic acid. It is found in plant-based sources such as chia, flax, and some nuts. ALA is not produced in the body.

- *EPA* stands for eicosapentaenoic acid. It is naturally found in the body but also comes from cold-water fish.
- *DHA* stands for docosahexaenoic acid. Just like EPA, it is found in the body and in cold-water fish. This compound works with the brain and nervous system. It has been studied as a potential memory support nutrient.

"Research shows that omega-3 fatty acids reduce inflammation and may help lower risk of chronic diseases such as heart disease, cancer, and arthritis. Omega-3 fatty acids are highly concentrated in the brain and appear to be important for cognitive (brain memory and performance) and behavioral function. Omega-3 fatty acids are considered essential fatty acids: They are necessary for human health but the body can't make them—you have to get them through food."[10]

Dr. William Penten Sears, the renowned pediatrician and diet expert of of AskDrSears.com states, "Fats can also influence brain development and performance, especially at either end of life—growing infants and elderly people. In fact, there are two windows of time in which the brain is especially sensitive to nutrition: the first two years of life for a growing baby and the last couple decades of life for a senior citizen. Both growing and aging brains need nutritious fat."[11]

The omega-3 fatty acid known as docosahexaenoic acid (DHA) is an important ingredient for optimal brain function. Earl Mindell, RPh, PhD, writes in *Earl Mindell's Supplement Bible*, "There's a reason why fish is known as brain food. It is a rich source of

---

10   University of Maryland Medical Center, "Omega-3 Fatty Acids," http://umm.edu/health/medical/altmed/supplement/omega3-fatty-acids#ixz-z2iaXVrSlv (Accessed 22 October 2013)

11   Dr. William Penten Sears, MD, Pediatrician, "Omega-3 And DHA As Brain Food" AskDrSears.com, http://www.askdrsears.com/topics/feeding-eating/family-nutrition/dha-and-omega-3s/dha-brain-food (Accessed 18 October 2013)

docosahexaenoic acid (DHA), a fatty acid that is found in high concentration in the gray matter of the brain. DHA is instrumental in the function of brain cell membranes, which are important for the transmission of brain signals."[12] By making cell membranes more fluid, omega-3 fatty acids, especially DHA, improve communication between the brain cells, according to *Mind Boosters* author Dr. Ray Sahelian, who states, "As a result, lack of omega-3 in the body can cause a communication breakdown in the brain, which is probably the last place you'd want such a breakdown to happen."[13]

In *Superfoods for Dummies*, Dr. Brent Agin and Shereen Jegtvig write, "Omega-3 fatty acids fight inflammation but they do so much more. They're particularly important for brain development and cognitive function, plus they may be important for eye health."[14]

When your aging uncle seems a little depressed or complains of "brain fog" it may be time to suggest that he increase his omega-3s as his balance of omega-6s vs omega-3s may be out of line. In addition, low levels of B vitamins are common among the elderly, writes Dr. Alan H. Pressman, DC, PH.C, C.C.N the author of *The Complete Idiot's Guide to Vitamins*.[15]

"Perhaps the most interesting research on omega-3 fatty acids involved their relationship to mental health ailments such as depression, attention deficit hyperactivity disorder, dementia, schizophrenia, bipolar disorder and Alzheimer's disease. Our brains

---

12   Dr. Earl Mindell, "Brain Health Dramatically Improved by Intake of Omega-3 Fatty Acids and Fish Oils," *Natural News*, http://www.naturalnews.com/016353_omega-3_fatty_acids_mental_health.html (Accessed October 18 2013)

13   Dr. Ray Sahelian, "Natural Brain Boosters," WebMD.com, http://www.webmd.com/balance/features/natural-brain-boosters?page=2 (Accessed 18 October 2013)

14   Dr. Brent Agin and Shereen Jegtvig, *Superfoods For Dummies*, (Wily Publishing Inc. 2009), 108

15   Dr. Alan H Pressman DC, PhD CCN and Sheila Buff, *The Complete Idiot's Guide to Vitamins And Minerals*, Third Edition, (Alpha Member of Penguin Group 2007), 62

are surprisingly fatty: over 60 percent of brain is fat. Omega-3 fatty acids promote the brain's ability to regulate mood-related signals. They are a crucial constituent of brain-cell membranes and are needed for normal nervous system function, mood regulation, and attention and memory functions"[16] writes the author of *SuperFoods RX* by Steven G. Pratt, MD and Kathy Matthews.

How can you combat or help prevent these maladies? Proper and complete nutrition is your key. By adjusting your lifestyle and consuming more fruits and vegetables you will be keeping your ratio of omega-6s and omega-3s in the proper proportions (always more 3 than 6). Most processed foods and some GMO foods feature omega-6 oils very heavily. Omega-6 is desirable in the food industry because of its very long shelf life. Omega-3 is found more in the fresh, unprocessed foods like chia seeds (and some other seeds), uncooked nuts (especially walnuts), fresh fish, winter squash, wild rice, and beans.

Make sure that the food you are consuming has enough B vitamins. Foods rich in the B family are: fish, meat, chicken, some dairy, nuts, beans, and dark green leafy vegetables. If you're in doubt, you can also use supplements to fill in any gaps.

If you are watching your weight, don't be led into the hype on how bad fats are. Just watch what kinds of fats you're eating. That's why you'll see real cream used in some of the MySeeds recipes. Real cream has the animal fat that's better for you than the chemicals and hydrogenated oils that can be in some of those diet whipped toppings.

Fats can also contribute to the level of satisfaction you have when eating a food. A fat-containing food item such as actual whipped cream usually brings satisfaction faster than artificial substitutes. When you're satisfied, you don't want to eat as much. Something that is lower in calories defeats its own purpose

16   Steven G. Pratt MD and Kathy Matthews, *SuperFoods RX—Fourteen Foods That Will Change Your Life*, (Harper 2005), 118

when you want to double the amount you're eating in order to find satisfaction.

A tablespoon of chia seeds contains nearly 2,500 milligrams of omega-3 fatty acids, plus the highest combined alpha-linolenic (ALA) and linoleic fatty acid percentage of all crops. As 2,100 milligrams, these numbers are equivalent to the omega-3s in three ounces of salmon. Yeah! No salmon smoothie for breakfast! How about a nice green apple chia omelet instead?

GREEN APPLE CHIA OMELET

Everyone knows that having a high-protein breakfast is a key to lasting energy and your fullness factor. If you eat a healthy breakfast that has fiber and protein, you won't be tempted to overeat at lunch or grab a snack between breakfast and lunch. Having an omelet in the morning will make those white-bread bagels or fried doubt nuts look much less appealing. As a change of pace from stir-fried veggies, have you tried half a green apple in your omelet? The little sweet crunchiness is fun and different. The apple peel gives you fiber. This is a quick, sunny way to start your day even if it *is* raining.

INGREDIENTS:

2 eggs
A splash of any type of milk
½ a sliced/chopped green apple
A small handful of low-fat shredded cheese
½ handful parsley
Black pepper to taste
A sprinkle of chia seeds

INSTRUCTIONS:

In a small bowl or measuring cup, fork-whisk the eggs and the milk. Precut the apple into thin slices as seen in the photo, and ready the cheese of choice. Coat a small skillet with cooking spray and heat the pan on medium for about thirty seconds. Pour in the mixed eggs. Cook for two to three minutes. Lift one side of the egg mixture so that any of the remaining uncooked egg run to the side of pan. Cook until no longer gelatinous. On one half of the omelet place the apple, parsley, cheese, and a couple of grinds of pepper, then sprinkle with a pinch of chia. Then fold the omelet over and serve a fresh new breakfast.

What about eggs and cholesterol? Years ago, eggs were thought to be a contributor to people's cholesterol levels. However, more recently this has been proven to be untrue. Dietary cholesterol only contributes to about 25 percent of a person's overall blood cholesterol levels, according to the American Heart Association.[17] The rest is made by your body and can be affected by family history and genetics. Aside from cholesterol, eggs also have protein, some healthy (unsaturated) fats, and many of the other vitamins and nutrients the body needs to stay healthy, such as vitamin B12, iron, vitamin A, and selenium.

Don't skip breakfast! "Your morning meal sets the stage for the way your blood sugar behaves the rest of the day," says Dr. Alicia Stanton, a women's health expert and anti-aging, integrative medicine practitioner. "If you skip it entirely, you deprive your brain and muscles of energizing glucose. Or if you grab a refined-carbohydrate meal, like a bagel, you'll experience a brief sugar spike but then inevitably crash." Then, "when insulin rushes in, it helps clear sugar, but it also sends the 'adrenal fatigue' signal to your adrenal glands to stop producing cortisol properly,"[18] endocrinologist Eva Cwynar, MD, author of *The Fatigue Solution* says.

---

17 American Heart Association, "About Cholesterol," http://www. heart.org/HEARTORG/Conditions/Cholesterol/AboutCholesterol/About-Cholesterol_UCM_001220_Article.jsp (Accessed 18 October 2013)

18 Dr. Alicia Stanton and Dr. Eva Cwynar, "9 Ways to Have More Energy," *Men's Health*, http://draliciastanton.com/tag/mens-health (Accessed 18 October 2013)

Fiber in the morning will help wake you up, let you feel less stressed, and keep away "brain fog." It is so simple to prepare a fruit and veggie smoothie or microwave quick oatmeal or a scrambled egg, and with the addition of chia, a complete protein, you will have created a wakeup call that may last all morning.

Chia as a Prebiotic and Probiotic

What are prebiotics and probiotics? Probiotics you've probably heard of because many yogurt companies love to advertise that their yogurt is loaded with these good bacteria. Yogurt, when properly prepared and stored, is a great source of good bacteria. Your body relies on good bacteria (called *flora*) in the stomach and intestines to properly break down foods. These good bacteria fight and crowd out the bad bacteria. This makes it easier for your immune system to help keep you healthy.

The book *Probiotics for Dummies* states that "70 to 90 percent of your immune system is located in the GI tract." And "good bacteria produce enzymes and proteins that can kill or inhibit harmful bacteria. In addition, the good guys secrete immunoglobulin A (an antibody), which fights infection,"[19] reports Dr. Shekhar Challa who is a board certified gastroenterologist.

Prebiotics are what the good bacteria eat. Good bacteria (and there are several strains, each of which helps you in different ways) love to feast on fresh veggies, soluble fiber, fermented foods such as yogurt and sauerkraut, green tea, and garlic.

The "bad bacteria" like animal fats, refined sugars, and flour. Bad bacteria produce unhelpful substances such as inflammatory particles, free radicals, excess gas, and acid. They can even produce toxins, which the liver and kidneys have to filter out later, making them work harder. Bad bacteria also have no problems letting

---

19   Dr. Shekhar Challa, *Probiotics for Dummies*, (John Wily & Sons Inc. 2012), 156 and 22–23

viruses thrive. Feed the good guys! They'll crowd out the bad when you feed them properly.

The first steps to better digestion and better microflora health are to eat enzyme-rich foods and chew your food properly to mix in the saliva. Saliva helps predigest your meal. The food then enters your stomach onto the next step of digestion. Jon Barron with *The Barron Report* and who serves on the Medical Advisory Board of the prestigious Health Sciences Institute, states this succinctly: "Only after this period of 'pre-digestion' are hydrochloric acid and pepsin introduced. The acid inactivates all of the food-based enzymes, but begins its own function of breaking down what is left of the meal in combination with the acid energized enzyme pepsin. Eventually, this nutrient-rich food concentrate moves on into the small intestine. Once this concentrate enters the small intestine, the acid is neutralized and the pancreas reintroduces digestive enzymes to the process. As digestion is completed, nutrients are passed through the intestinal wall and into the bloodstream."[20]

Have you read that heat destroys food enzymes? Heating destroys some enzymes and it kills bacteria too, both good and bad. You'll find that in many of our recipes we use lightly cooked or not-cooked-at-all veggies and fruits. We add yogurt to many recipes to get that lower-fat-but-still-creamy taste. We love live-culture yogurt as it has about a bazillion of the "good guys" to repopulate positive microflora for you. However, they are delicate and don't like heat. Therefore, stirring yogurt into a warm sauce just killed your "good team." Heat doesn't really affect the function of fiber, though, so you don't have to worry as much about heating your prebiotics.

All throughout human history, we have found that fermented foods have increased healthy digestion. These include fermented cabbage (e.g., sauerkraut and some types of Korean cabbage),

---

20   John Barron, "Stomach Acid, Baseline of Health Foundation" http://www.jonbarron.org/article/stomach-acid (Accessed 18 October 2013)

nattō (fermented soybean), and yogurt. Low-fat yogurt will help with your cholesterol levels and is an excellent source of calcium. Yogurt has very little lactose (milk sugar), which disagrees with some people's digestive system (i.e., lactose-intolerant people). Ancient humans didn't understand why but knew that it just worked. Different types of probiotic bacteria (different strains) do different things and can help with different conditions. It's important to look up which strain could help you the best.

Antibiotics and aging will also affect your gut flora. Antibiotics kill most bacteria—the good and bad. So if you must take an antibiotic treatment, once it is complete, start repopulating your gut with the "good guys." Many health food and vitamin shops carry a "shot" of mixed good bacteria. And it is especially important to the elderly to keep their "good guys" active and healthy. Preventative maintenance for the elderly will help fight off infections and frailty.

Put a sprinkle of chia into your breakfast or snack yogurt so that your "new good guys" have some fiber to make them happy. The good bacteria will feast and grow.

PREBIOTICS

While probiotics are the actual microflora that help you digest foods, prebiotics are the foods that they like to eat. When you keep your microflora fed and healthy, they'll help protect you. Prebiotics are generally fiber, but especially soluble fiber. They serve as food for good bacteria. You can't digest or absorb nutrients from either soluble or insoluble fiber; however, your good bacteria can. When you eat foods such as bananas, barley, garlic, oats, onions, tofu, and chia you are feeding the good guys.

Dr. Challa, author of *Probiotics for Dummies* writes, "When you ingest prebiotic fiber, the fermentation that takes place in your gut helps with water and electrolyte reabsorption and produces short-chain fatty acids (SCFAs), which help maintain the lining of the bowel. Fiber can be water insoluble or water soluble. Bacteria in the gut ferment less than 50 percent of water-insoluble fiber, whereas water-soluble fiber is fermented well by your gut microbiota."[21] So, feed your team of good guys with the soluble fiber you can actually see on the outside of each chia seed!

CHIA CHICKEN CAESAR-ISH SALAD

This fresh and easy riff on a Caesar salad will up your probiotics and your veggie count for the day. Because it is so filling with the addition of whole-wheat pasta, chia, and chicken, you won't need to worry about "just having a salad" for dinner. Hopefully there will be a little left over so that you can pack it in a pita pocket for lunch. This makes two-plus servings. Yum.

INGREDIENTS:
FOR THE SALAD:
   2 chicken breasts, grilled or broiled
   About 6 oz cooked whole wheat pasta
   3 plum tomatoes
   Several large handfuls of mixed greens of your choice
   A large handful of broccoli slaw
   ½ a package of frozen artichoke hearts, thawed
   Sprinkle of shredded cheese of your choice (cheddar shown here)

FOR THE DRESSING:
   ¼ cup plain nonfat yogurt
   2 tablespoons low-fat olive oil mayonnaise

---

21   Dr. Shekhar Challa, *Probiotics for Dummies*, (John Wily & Sons Inc. 2012), 33

1 tablespoon red wine vinegar

1 clove garlic, minced

1 tablespoon Dijon mustard

2 tablespoons parmesan/Romano cheese, grated

1 teaspoon lemon juice

A couple drops of Worcestershire sauce

2 tablespoons chia gel

Fresh black pepper to taste

INSTRUCTIONS:

Grill or broil the chicken breasts and set aside. Prepare the pasta according to the package directions. Drain and run under cool water. Place the pasta, thawed artichoke hearts, sliced plum tomatoes, and broccoli slaw in a bowl. Combine all the dressing ingredients in a small bowl, stir, and do a taste test so that you know how much fresh black pepper to add. Toss to coat the pasta mixture. Plate the greens and place the pasta mixture on top. Slice the chicken and place that on top. Dress with cheese shreds if desired.

Note: Artichoke hearts, yogurt, and aged parmesan/Romano cheese all deliver probiotics that will feed your good flora in the gut. We bet you are feeling an energy surge just reading this recipe!

CHIA MELON BERRY SPLASH!

INGREDIENTS:

1 banana

½ cup milk of choice

2 handfuls of fresh spinach

1 cup prepared strawberries

1 cup cantaloupe chunks

1 teaspoon grated ginger root

1 tablespoon dry Chia seeds

1 lime, zested and juiced (or 2 tablespoons lime juice.)

DIRECTIONS:

In your blender place the milk and spinach. Blend to chop the leaves to a tiny bite size consistency. Add the remaining ingredients and blend.

RASPBERRY POACHED CHIA CHICKEN SALAD

Raspberry vinegar is the key to this nearly sweet but slightly zingy fruit salad. Loaded with protein and veggies, you will think, "Wow! I can stick with this sort of healthy eating." With "orange-ed" brown rice on the bottom, this salad is both filling and loaded with so much of the nutrition your body craves. This salad will serve four.

INGREDIENTS:

    3 small chicken breasts
    ¼ cup plus 1 tablespoon raspberry balsamic vinegar
    ⅓ cup low-fat plain yogurt
    1 dash cayenne pepper
    ¼ cup chopped red onion
    1 box of frozen artichoke hearts
    1 cup of uncooked brown rice (makes 2 cups when cooked)
    2 tablespoons chia, divided (1 tablespoon for the rice and 1 for the yogurt dressing)
    1 kiwi
    1 avocado
    1 large naval orange
    Handful of raspberries
    Nuts or seeds of your choice

INSTRUCTIONS:

Start by zesting and sectioning the orange while reserving the juice. Start the brown rice cooking per the directions on the package. Add a tablespoon of chia and the orange juice. Simmer for the allotted time. Cool to room temperature and add the zest.

Defrost the artichoke hearts.

Next, in a large skillet with a lid, poach the chicken breasts in one-quarter cup of raspberry vinegar. Cooking times will vary, but it should be about seven minutes on each side. Cool the chicken and shred it into bite-size pieces.

In a bowl, place the chicken shreds, yogurt, chia, red onion, and the remaining one tablespoon of vinegar.

Place the cooled rice on the bottom of the plate. Next, add your greens of choice with just a sprinkle of vinegar on the greens, and then place the chicken mixture on top. Garnish with the berries, artichoke halves, kiwi, and avocado wedges, and top off with nuts or seeds of choice.

Note: If raspberries aren't available, thin slices of pineapple work great too!

Chia and Nutrition

Nutrition has two forms: macronutrients and micronutrients. Macronutrients include protein, carbohydrates, and fats. Protein provides energy and the building blocks for muscle cells; carbohydrates are an easy, ready form of energy that can also be stored for later; and fats help maintain cell walls, convert into energy, and aid in the absorption of certain vitamins that you need to stay healthy. Chia contains plant protein and healthy omega-3 oil (a healthy fat).

Micronutrients are vitamins, minerals, and other compounds that your body requires only very small amounts of. These can also be referred to as "trace minerals."

Micronutrients include

- Sodium (regulates the fluid balance in your cells)
- Manganese (promotes bone formation and helps you use the energy from fats)
- Chloride (regulates electrolytes and helps maintain proper pH levels in cells)

- Iodine (promotes healthy thyroid function and helps metabolize fats)
- Magnesium (helps the heart maintain a normal rhythm and so much more)
- Vitamins A, B, C, D, E, and K
- Iron (is used for making red blood cells that oxygenate all your other organs)
- Boron (works together with calcium to build and maintain bone mass; it's especially important for all people later on in life to help avert arthritis and the symptoms of menopause and andropause; it also helps your cell walls stay strong)
- Selenium (helps the body make antioxidants)
- Choline (is important for brain health, preventing fatty liver, and promoting artery health)

You already know that chia seeds are nutritious, but did you know which micronutrients they contain? Chia has boron, all of the B vitamins, vitamin C, and calcium. How can trace minerals help you stay healthy? Find out about the wealth of trace minerals that are all around you in different tasty foods.

TRACE MINERALS: TINY AMOUNTS FOR BIG HEALTH RESULTS

Everyone knows that good health is associated with getting enough vitamins and minerals, but do you know about trace minerals? These special substances are often overlooked because you need them only in such small amounts. However, it's a *big* mistake to leave them out of your diet because, as you'll soon see, trace minerals may be small, but they're super effective at keeping you healthy.

Which minerals are trace minerals? Trace minerals include iron, manganese, zinc, copper, iodine, chromium, boron, and selenium.

You'll find some of these on the periodic table, but you can also find them in many healthy foods. The amounts you need are very small, only milligrams or micrograms, and it's important to not get too much as well. Maintaining a balance is important, especially for minerals. For example, getting too much zinc will interfere with your ability to absorb iron and copper, and too much iron results in free radicals and oxidative damage. (Free radicals help cause premature signs of aging.)

Where do trace minerals come from? Trace minerals can be found in many foods, including raw vegetables, nuts, seeds, some fruits, and certain meats. However, it is important to keep in mind that many foods today are *not* as healthy as they once were! Beef that's factory farmed is often nutrient deficient. Cows who feed on a proper natural diet of grasses (and not expired candy, wood sawdust, corn, animal meat, and cheap grain, which you'll often find used today) have much better quality and healthier meat. They pass on the nutrients found in the grass to you, so choosing grass-fed meats is a big advantage. You'll find trace minerals such as iron and manganese here.

Vegetables and fruits suffer similarly, as the land used to grow them may be depleted from years of repeated farming and use of chemical fertilizers. Food labels aren't required to document the soil history of, say, a tomato or your fresh broccoli. The items will look the same, but something important may be missing! It's important to ask your doctor about your own personal mineral levels to see if they're where they should be for optimal health.

What do trace minerals do for you?

- Chromium and manganese: These minerals work together to help you properly process carbohydrates. Manganese also works with bone formation and keeps bones strong.

- Zinc: This is important for immune and reproductive health. However, too much zinc can actually interfere with your ability to fight off disease.
- Copper: Helps you use iron properly and aids with cartilage growth and repair.

With all these great benefits coming from such small amounts of minerals, how can you be sure you're getting enough? Turning to unusual (at least to Westernized diets) foods can be a big help. Sea vegetables are rich in trace minerals because the ocean has not been nutritionally depleted as some soils have. Free-range and grass-fed meats, as previously mentioned, can also be a good source, as well as cold-water fish. However, what if seaweed and algae aren't a part of your menu? What if you don't like the idea of harming animals or the taste of fish?

You can still turn to plants for good taste and good nutrition.

Local farms and small farms (farmers markets) usually use land that hasn't been overfarmed, so they're a good place to start. Another easy tip is making your plate as colorful as possible. By selecting a wide variety of very different colored foods, you're usually also selecting foods with a great range of micronutrients. Don't overlook nuts and seeds They may be small, but did you know that Brazil nuts, cashews, almonds, and chestnuts have a lot of potassium and phosphorus? Seeds and grains such as quinoa have calcium, pumpkin seeds have magnesium, and chia seeds have more calcium by weight than milk and more iron than spinach and include boron, the trace mineral, to help you absorb it all. If you throw in complete protein, like that found in meat, as well as healthy omega-3 oils, like those in fish, you've got a real winner.

Why has chia escaped the nutrition loss that overfarmed foods suffer from? It grows in places that are hot and dry where you can't raise traditional crops. These rough conditions have forced the plant to be hardy and resourceful, using everything from the soil around it. This soil still has the trace minerals and ordinary minerals (e.g., calcium) that you require.

Just because trace minerals are so small doesn't mean they should be overlooked. These tiny amounts of minerals have a big job to perform in the body. There's one mineral in particular that's so special you'll definitely want to know more about it.

WHAT MINERAL CAN HELP PREVENT TWENTY-TWO DIFFERENT CONDITIONS?

What mineral is so important that hospitals feel the need to keep it on hand in case of emergencies? The answer is magnesium, and its importance is often overlooked. Even though it's so vital to good health, how often do you hear about it? It's thought to be because magnesium is a natural substance. It occurs naturally in foods and in mineral deposits but that also means that it's not very profitable to sell. It's not a prescription drug and it's not synthesized in some factory for big money.

Doctors say that magnesium deficiency can trigger twenty-two different conditions such as diabetes, migraines, or irregular heart-beats. Some conditions are irritating (e.g., leg cramps at night), while others, such as being extra susceptible to kidney disease, are quite serious. Magnesium helps the body absorb calcium and helps repair cell membranes. There are so many great reasons to ensure you have enough magnesium in your diet, but how do you know if you're getting enough?

If you like foods such as walnuts, cashews, other tree nuts, shrimp, broccoli, and leafy green vegetables, you're likely getting more magnesium than most people. But how many times per week are you eating one serving of them? Processed foods, white flour, and eating the meat of animals with poor diets won't give anyone any magnesium, but all of those not-so-good-for-you items are so common and easy to get today. But what if you're allergic to nuts or shrimp? What if you don't want a salad of leafy greens every night? There are other options to consider, and they're both inexpensive and easy.

The first is the chia seed, which has fifteen times more magnesium than broccoli, and, unlike broccoli, you can make the seed taste like anything you want.

The second way to healthy magnesium levels is through supplementation. With depleted soil for crops, even the known magnesium-rich foods have lower levels of it today than they did twenty years ago. Magnesium citrate and magnesium aspartate are the two easiest-to-absorb forms of this great mineral. They're also inexpensive for capsules with a few hundred milligrams each. Even if you are eating chia seeds each day, you might want to consider a supplement as well. Having your magnesium levels tested by a doctor is a great first step toward better health. Don't wait for a problem to arrive in your life before taking active and safe steps to stay healthy.

Magnesium supplementation is also important because certain foods can actually take magnesium out of your body. Alcohol, coffee, certain sodas, and having unbalanced levels of sodium and potassium (i.e., an excess of salt) can all lower your levels of magnesium. You can easily see why the foods available today lead many people to becoming magnesium deficient. It's still all right to enjoy the magnesium-lowering foods in moderation, just make sure you supplement with a good-quality magnesium capsule.

WHY ARE VEGETABLES LOSING THEIR NUTRITION? FIND OUT NOW AND SAVE YOUR HEALTH!

If you've heard it once, you've heard it a zillion times. "If you want to be healthy, eat your vegetables!" Certainly, this is still good advice, but there's a problem creeping in. Vegetables and fruits are losing their nutritious qualities. They may not be providing you with the healthy kick they used to. Sure they look the same, and they might even taste the same, but did you know. "You'd have to eat ten servings of spinach to get the same level of minerals from just one serving about fifty years ago."[22] That's what Elmer Heinrich found out when he did his research for his book *The Root of All Disease*. It's amazing, but it's also terrible, because no one is ever going to eat ten servings of spinach in one day. To get your optimum nutrition, according these new statistics, you'd have to be an elephant! Or at least eat as much as one.

But why is all this happening? It sounds rather farfetched at first that a vegetable or fruit could look and taste the same, but be so lacking in nutrients you need. However, there are several reasons which most people would never think of. It's important to know the cause behind something as vital as your own nutrition. You try to eat right, you try to have your required servings of fruits and vegetables each day—but what are they really doing for you?

Overfarming causes depleted soil: Despite farmers' best efforts with chemical fertilizers and crop rotations, the huge human population's demands on the soil causes overfarming. Nutrients you need are depleted from the soil by hundreds of previous crop cycles—and if they're not there, the plants can't absorb them. This is especially true for the trace minerals we all need to maintain good health.

Crops are now being bred for the wrong thing: Fruits and veggies are chosen for several reasons, none of which is their nutritional value. The important thing about them is how they look, how long they stay fresh, how much they weigh, and how they can resist weeds and pests. Are any of those factors helping *your* health? No, they're just helping the bottom line. These are no "frankenfoods," either (genetically modified crops); they're your

---

22   Elmer Heinrich, *The Root of All Disease*, http://nutrilife.com.my/go/ elmerheinrich/root_of_all_disease.pdf page 45 , (Accessed 22 October 2013)

usual 100 percent natural crops which have gone through selective breeding for money making, *not* nutritional qualities. Sure, some genetically modified crops, such as the black tomato, are super nutritious, but they're still years away from a real market release.

An experiment for you: If you look around on TV, do you see commercials for "grow-at-home tomatoes"? Have you ever enjoyed a tomato from a vine at a friend or neighbor's house? These homegrown fruits (yes, a tomato is a fruit) often taste *much* better than the ones you find in the supermarket. That's why kits and vines are so popular in gardens. Supermarket tomatoes are raised only to look good, stay fresh, and make the high "weight grade." They're *not* bred for taste or nutrition quality.

It's easy to demonstrate this with something like a tomato, because they have a specific flavor that everyone recognizes and are easy to grow at home in many climates—unlike spinach or peaches. The point is that this type of "all style, no substance" is afflicting more than tomatoes and affecting much more than flavor.

These statistics show various losses from 1975 compared to 2001. The US Department of Agriculture (USDA) came up with the facts and *Life Extension Magazine* is quoted on the following statistics:[23]

- Apples: vitamin A is down 41 percent
- Broccoli: calcium and vitamin A are down 50 percent
- Cauliflower: vitamin C is down 45 percent, vitamin B1 is down 48 percent, and vitamin B2 is down 47 percent

That's a big drop, and other fruits and vegetables are also affected to varying degrees. So, what can you do about it? You want to eat healthy to stay healthy, so taking action in your diet is a step to

---

23   *Life Extension Magazine*, "Dirt Poor: Have Fruits and Vegetables Become Less Nutritious?," *Scientific American*, http://www.scientificamerican. com/article.cfm?id=soil-depletion-and-nutrition-loss (Accessed 18 October 2013)

take right away. Vitamin supplements are a great idea. Because vitamins are made, not grown, they are held to nutritional standards, and must contain exactly what you see on the label. But, one cannot live on pills alone! First, consider organic foods and using a home garden. Chances are, your yard was never the site of a huge company farm featuring depleted soil. The foods you grow at home can still pick up necessary minerals from your soil.

But what about apartment or condo dwellers in the city? No time for a garden? As a next choice, small farms and local growers are also more likely to be farming on land that is not nutritionally deficient or using "maximum-shelf-life" variety plants. Local farms don't have to ship long distance and they know you'll be back for more if you like their produce's *flavor*.

Another easy solution is the chia seed, of course. Chia plants grow only in areas most other plants hate. You couldn't grow a peach or an apple where chia likes to grow. It only grows where it's hot and dry all the time. This means that the land used to grow chia hasn't already been stripped of nutrients. Worried about pesticides? Don't be. The plant takes care of itself like no other by producing an oil in the leaves and stems that insects and other pests can't stand. Chemical pesticides don't even need to be touched when you've got chia growing. The plants are still pulling in all the nutrients you need while being free from toxic chemical pesticides.

So by looking to a food that's unusual and new, you can still get the nutrients your body needs despite depleted soil in many areas. Don't let these startling statistics stop you on your quest for greater health, energy, and longevity. You can still take control of your nutrition and improve your health.

ANTIOXIDANTS FOR ANTI-AGING

When you think of anti-aging, do you think of expensive creams, spa treatments, or surgery?

If so, you might want to look at another less expensive and healthier alternative: food. Certain foods can do much more than fight the outward signs of aging, they can also help ward off inner symptoms as well. Many problems of the body are caused by inflammation and oxidative damage done by free radicals. If you can fight these two causes, you can look and feel better. The foods you eat provide your body with the power to fight damage and inflammation, especially when you mix different foods together. Antioxidants should be a part of your nutrition consideration each day.

What are free radicals? These bad molecules can be a byproduct of normal metabolism. Free radical damage can also be caused by exposure to pollutants in your environment, food, or drink. Everyone is exposed to free radicals as a part of daily life, so it's important to know what they do and how you can minimize their effects on you.

Free radicals are formed when a molecule has an unpaired electron and becomes unstable. When a molecule is unstable, it will steal an electron from the nearest item it encounters (usually a cell in your body). Then, the molecule that was robbed becomes a free radical itself, scavenging for a spare electron to use so that it will be stable again. Free radicals can damage almost anything they come into contact with, which is why the immune system sometimes creates them and uses them as a weapon against invaders it deems harmful.

Because free radicals can create chain reactions by stealing electrons from the molecules that make up your cells, they can cause inflammation, cell damage, and signs of early aging. It's in your best interest to fight free radicals with antioxidants. The best way to get your antioxidants is to eat them. Because you really "are what you eat," the right foods supply lots of free radical fighters.

You can fight free radicals with lots of different foods. Food is your most potent weapon against free radical damage. Certain foods and compounds in them have the building blocks your body is looking for as it stops free radicals in their tracks. There are many different compounds in natural foods that fight free radicals. They do this by having a spare electron available to lend. When one of these unstable free radicals approaches an antioxidant, the antioxidant gives up its extra electron and neutralizes the danger. An antioxidant doesn't become unstable because that extra electron was always just a spare. When you have plenty of free radical fighting supplies "in stock," your body is able to deal with these bad guys right away. They don't get a chance to damage cells.

What are the most common antioxidants you can look for in foods?

Anthocyanins: These powerful helpers are the dark pigments in plants. Plants will add anthocyanins to certain items in order to give them a rich, dark color. Things like blueberries, blackberries, purple cabbage, cherries, and pomegranates all have plenty of anthocyanins. Pale foods such as cauliflower, white potatoes, and lima beans don't have any. There are even some exotic foods such as purple potatoes, heirloom tomatoes (these may have streaks of dark red, purple, and orange), and black chia seeds with dark, rich colors for you to choose.

Betatene: This is what gives beets a dark, red color. It's more potent than polyphenols, which are found in green tea, black tea, dark chocolate, and olive oil. Don't discount polyphenols, though; green tea has earned its reputation as a health drink for many reasons. (Note: drinking raw beet root juice may lower blood pressure in people who have hypertension. If you're going to drink it and are on medication for blood pressure, you may want to have your doctor watch over your progress.)

Vitamins A and C: These vitamins are also antioxidants. Most people know the benefits of these fat and water-soluble vitamins but overlook their property as free radical fighters as well. Fruits and vegetables are rich in A and C. Paprika, dried parsley, cayenne, chili powder, and basil are all seasonings loaded with A. Citrus fruits, kiwis, peppers, leafy greens, guavas, papayas, and even strawberries have lots of vitamin C.

Antioxidants work best when they're mixed together. Taking a supplement of an isolated antioxidant generally isn't as effective as mixing together multiples in one meal. They all work with each other and build on each other's benefits. Notice how tomatoes have both vitamin C and anthocyanins. Adding seasonings to your food, such as a tasty basil pesto, diced peppers in chili, or parsley in tabbouleh, not only makes the food taste better but makes it healthier as well.

The less commonly known but still important antioxidants of chia are myricetin, quercetin, kaempferol, caffeic acid, and chlorogenic acid. Did you know that quercetin is known for its naturally occurring antihistamine and anti-inflammatory effects and its ability to help reduce LDL (the bad cholesterol)? Chlorogenic acid requires more study but so far looks like it has an anti-diabetic effect and a blood-sugar balancing effect, and some people feel it helps their weight loss efforts.

Antioxidants and citrus zest: Have you noticed lots of recipes throughout this book contain citrus zest from oranges, limes, or lemons? Not only does zest really freshen up the flavor of your recipes, it's really great for you too! Citrus peels contain high levels of antioxidants. As antioxidants, citrus peels may contribute to the protection of your DNA from cancer-causing damage. According to *Medicinal Herbs and Spices*,[24] citrus peels contain greater amounts of antioxidants than vitamin E. When used in their natural form, the antioxidant effects of citrus peels are enhanced by the high levels of vitamin C found in citrus fruits. That's why you so often see zesting, sectioning, or juicing of great citrus flavors in our recipes.

---

24   Angela Stokes, "Citrus Peel Benefits," Livestrong.com, http://www. livestrong.com/article/155590-citrus-peel-benefits/ (Accessed 18 October 2013)

What is the ORAC score? If you've looked into antioxidants before, you might have run into the word *ORAC*. ORAC stands for oxygen radical absorbency capacity, or the scientific measurement of the antioxidant value of a food. The higher this score, the more free radical fighting power the food involved possesses. Currently, the USDA recommends a diet of fruits and vegetables that will allow you to consume between 3,000 to 5,000 ORAC units per day.

What foods are high on the ORAC table?

- Chia seed (soaked)
- Unsweetened cocoa powder
- Acai berry
- Prunes (drying the fruit condenses the nutrients and the sugars)
- Raisins
- Blueberries
- Blackberries
- Kale
- Cranberries
- Strawberries
- Raspberries
- Pomegranates
- Spinach, raw
- Brussels sprouts
- Alfalfa sprouts
- Spinach, steamed
- Broccoli florets
- Beets
- Red bell pepper
- Onion

The list above goes from roughly highest to lowest. You'll also find that spices are very high in ORAC value. However, no one eats as much of a spice as they do of a fruit or a vegetable. Fruits and veggies are foods you eat in quantity, so it's OK that they fall lower on the ORAC scale than very small, intense spices. Every little bit adds up to free radical fighting for you. Why are there no numbers in the list above? The ORAC value of foods can change based on how they're prepared and stored. Different companies can test foods with different methods and get different scores too. This list is just an average of several different scores for each of the items. For instance, there may be some debate about whether the blueberry beats the blackberry on the chart, while the following week you could see the cranberry versus the raspberry.

Precise numbering isn't as important as eating delicious, healthy berries and fresh fruits and greens.

Antioxidants are easier to add to your diet because they tend to be found in delicious foods that lots of people already like. Dark-colored, appealing sweet berries, bright, colorful peppers, fruity plums, peaches, and nectarines—all of these seasonal treats are antioxidant rich. The main consideration for antioxidants is just to be sure to eat a variety of colorful fruits and vegetables. A rainbow on the plate not only looks good and tastes good, it's better for you too. These easy recipes can help you get started.

CHIA DARK FRUITS ANTIOXIDANT SALAD OR SIDE

As you have read, deeply colored fruits and veggies have the most antioxidants (anthocyanins) and this salad is absolutely loaded with them! This little dressing is refreshing and puts a little zing to the fruit flavors. If you would like to make this into a side dish, just add more dark greens and a cup of cooked and chilled orzo.

INGREDIENTS:
FOR THE DRESSING:
¼ cup raspberries or strawberries (defrosted works fine)
1 tablespoon olive oil

1 tablespoon chia gel

2 tablespoons raspberry vinegar

2 tablespoons minced red onion

A sliver of jalapeño, minced (you decide how much heat you want)

1 garlic clove, smashed and minced

FOR THE SALAD:

Dark greens of your choice (baby spinach has a very mild flavor)

1 plum (the darker, the better)

½ cup papaya chunks (or cantaloupe)

Raspberries or strawberries

Pomegranate arils* (optional)

INSTRUCTIONS:

First, make the easy dressing. In a food processor or mini chopper, add your fresh or defrosted raspberries or strawberries. Puree until smooth. Then add all of the other dressing ingredients and puree again. Set this aside in the fridge for about ten minutes so that the pepper can add its heat while the chia blends the flavors together.

For the salad, choose your favorite dark greens. We like baby spinach because it is so mild that even kids can be convinced to eat it. It's not going to interfere with the sweet tastes of these great fruits. Cut the plum and papaya into bite-sized pieces. If you're using strawberries, make sure to clean them well, then cut into bite-size pieces. Pomegranates aren't always in season. However, they're a super-powerful antioxidant fruit when they are in season, so make sure to sprinkle on some sweet, tart arils if you can find a pomegranate in your local grocery.

Place all ingredients in your salad bowl and dress with the fruity dressing and you're ready to serve.

*The small translucent kernels found inside a pomegranate are called arils. Each one is full of fiber and tasty juice. Inside each aril is a small white edible soft seed.

FIESTA BOWL CHIA DINNER

This is a fiesta of color on your plate. This meal is loaded with fresh yellow mango, red tomato, purple Spanish onion, and cool green avocado and then spiced up with jalapeño. Vibrant colors of fruits and vegetables indicate that you are getting the nutrition your body requires to provide long-lasting energy.

When you are removing the flesh from the avocado, be sure to get the vivid green layer next to the skin, as extra nutrients are stored there.* This recipe is quick and easy, especially if you have brown rice saved in advance for this party-in-your-mouth dinner!

INGREDIENTS:
   1 mango
   1 medium avocado
   1 tomato
   ¼-inch round of Spanish onion
   1 cup cooked brown rice
   1 cup shredded chicken
   1 cup black beans (canned)
   Lots of greens of your choice
   ½ tablespoon minced jalapeño pepper
   1 dash red pepper flakes
   1 clove garlic, smashed and minced
   2 tablespoons lime juice
   2 tablespoons chia gel
   2 teaspoons lemon juice

INSTRUCTIONS:
First, cook the rice according to the package directions. Then, while the rice cooks, drain and rinse the canned black beans. If you're using precooked rotisserie chicken, simply shred into

bite-size pieces and sprinkle with lemon juice and pepper flakes. Or, microwave a quartered chicken breast in a glass dish until no longer pink inside. Let cool, then shred into bite-size pieces.

Remove the skin and cut up the mango, avocado, and tomato into bite-size cubes. Then, dice the onion and mince the jalapeño pepper. Place these fruits and vegetables in a large bowl and stir in the lime juice. If you like a hotter dish, you can always add more pepper. However, if you're adding more jalapeño, be careful if you plan to have any leftovers as the dish will get hotter as it stands.

When the rice is done cooking, stir the beans into the hot rice to warm them and add the chia gel. To assemble your fiesta bowls, first lay down a layer of greens. Then place the bean and rice mixture on top. Scoop the fruit and veggie mixture over the warm rice and top with the chicken shreds. This makes three to four dinners. It also depends on the size and amount of fruits and vegetables you add.

*Don't be afraid of the avocado! It has been called a fatty food in the media but you'll be amazed by what the healthy fats will do for you! When you put avocado in a salad, it increases absorption of carotenoids from the salad between 200 to 400 percent. If that amazing increase wasn't enough for you, there are phytosterols, which fight inflammation, and oleic acid, which helps the digestive system, much like olive oil. So not only do avocados provide a light mild flavor and great nutrition on their own; they actually boost the nutritional power of the healthy foods you pair them with!

DECADENT DARK CHOCOLATE HEALTH POPSICLE
A popsicle that's actually good for you? Amazing!

This cool treat has absolutely nothing in it that's bad for you. There are zero added sugars so you can enjoy this popsicle at any time without guilt. Unsweetened baking cocoa powder makes this pop very chocolaty but not too sweet. It's great for you too, so you can enjoy it at any time of the day, even for breakfast!

Regular unsweetened baking cocoa will make a fudgy, textured, delightful popsicle. Bananas don't ever freeze completely. They have a creamy texture when frozen so when you add chocolate, the pop turns out fudgy. Cocoa labeled "extra dark" or "specialty dark" and sometimes "Dutched dark" will create pops that are nearly black in color and have a less sweet, very cacao-type flavor. However, keep in mind that the Dutch processing takes away a little bit of the antioxidant content of the chocolate.

INGREDIENTS:
  1 banana
  1 teaspoon chia seeds
  1 ½ tablespoon unsweetened baking cocoa
  2 tablespoons rice milk

INSTRUCTIONS:
In a food processor or blender, combine all ingredients until a smooth puree forms. Now you're ready to scoop into your molds. If the banana is especially large, the mixture can become extra thick so you can add another tablespoon of milk to thin it to a pourable consistency.

The banana adds all the sweetness you'll need for this popsicle. You know that unsweetened baking chocolate can be bitter on its own, but the banana here really has the power to make it sweet and wonderful. Rice milk, almond milk, or soy milk can be used. These are not acid forming and are free of added hormones. This treat may be simple but it's a real winner!

Note: Dark chocolate (as a snack by itself) is actually good for you too. Low in fat, the pure dark stuff (in small amounts) is also thought to reduce bad, or LDL, cholesterol and is packed with antioxidants. If you are craving chocolate and want a piece of chocolate instead of this popsicle, choose really dark chocolate—ideally 70 percent cacao or higher—that doesn't have a lot of extras such as milk and sugar added to it. The additives reduce the health benefits of the chocolate.

Chia for Vegetarians

Vegetarianism can be a great, healthy way of eating. You avoid hormones found in most meats, it's environmentally friendlier than eating meat, and it's much easier to avoid unhealthy fats. However, because meat does have some B vitamins, complete protein, amino acids, and several other health essentials, missing out on meat means that you need to take a variety of vegetables, seeds, nuts, legumes, beans, and grains into consideration. You can get these essentials from the plant world but you need to keep an eye on your menu.

THINKING ABOUT GOING VEGETARIAN BUT WORRIED ABOUT PROTEIN?

Are you already living the vegetarian lifestyle? If so, you've no doubt considered the protein issue. The human body needs protein to survive and thrive. For most people that protein comes from meat and when you stop eating it you've got to think of other choices. Many plant sources such as nuts, seeds, and soy products provide some. But then you're faced with having to eat a certain thing every day or risk getting sick.

It's a serious consideration for any vegetarian. Most of the plant proteins are incomplete, meaning you have to combine foods—eating certain things together in order to properly replicate inside the body the protein found in animal sources. And what if you don't like tofu? Not everyone is going to like it and it has such a reputation of being "essential" in the vegetarian lifestyle that it keeps many people from ever trying to become vegetarian. Plus, emerging studies concluding that too much soy isn't good for men further puts the issue on the fence.

The discovery of chia seeds and their complete protein will help any vegetarian achieve a proper amount of complete protein and make the lifestyle more attractive to any carnivore who is considering it. More tofu recipes? A new way to eat beans? No!

Chia seeds have complete protein; you don't have to combine them with other foods. That's uncommon in the plant world. Chia is 23 percent protein by weight. Without the soy estrogens, it's safe for men to consume any amount. The chia plant is also grown without pesticides, so making chia seeds does not harm insects or the environment. It truly is a "green" food! The plant makes an oil in its stems and leaves that insects and other pests can't stand, so there's no need for harsh chemicals. It is also one of the few plant sources that provides complete protein like that found in meat.

For vegetarians, omega-3 oil is also an issue. Its primary source is in fish. Omega-3–rich diets adopted by cultures who eat a lot of fish, such as the Japanese and Greek Islanders, have been proven to reduce heart disease risk, lower cholesterol, and lessen arthritis. However, if you don't want to sacrifice eating fish or even if you don't like the idea of eating fish many days of the week, chia seeds are the answer once again.

Chia is rich in omega-3 oil as well as calcium. In fact, it has six times the calcium (by weight) as milk. With chia seed in the house you won't have to worry about harming the ocean or eating fishy flavors. With the oceans in danger and some of the fish even absorbing poisons, now is the right time to turn to alternate omega-3 sources.

You don't have to be afraid to try vegetarianism and if you're already eating the vegetarian way, chia will make it so much easier for you to get your essential nutrients while continuing to enjoy the foods you love. Take advantage of easy, delicious, complete protein right now, with chia seeds!

VEGETARIAN MEN: SHOULD YOU BEWARE THE SECRETS OF SOY YOU'RE NOT BEING TOLD ABOUT?

Soy and soy products have come under closer inspection in the news lately. If you've taken a look and if you're a vegetarian or are investigating the vegetarian eating style, you've likely seen that the news isn't all good. Men especially have cause for concern because of the high plant-estrogen content of the soy bean and plant. Before reaching for another block of tofu or taking a closer look at the vegetarian diet, there are a few things you should know.

First of all, why is this especially a *men's* issue? Everyone has a little bit of both types of hormones: testosterone and estrogen. They play important roles in the body's many functions. Men have more testosterone than estrogen and they don't need any more than the body already produces. Declining testosterone production in older men causes health problems as the testosterone-estrogen balance is then upset. Testosterone levels in boys are also important for proper development and bone health. Adding extra estrogen into the mix isn't a good idea at any stage.

So what's the problem with soy? It has high levels of plant estrogens. *Plant estrogens* are hormones the plant uses for its daily function. They're not the same as the ones found in humans, and, if consumed, are one thousand times *less* effective than human hormones. They are sometimes called *phytoestrogens* or *lignans*.

But as a vegetarian or anyone trying to adopt a healthy eating pattern, soy and soy products often play a big role. Don't want nasty bovine hormones? Drink soy milk. Don't want to hurt animals by eating meat? Get protein from tofu blocks, tofu dogs, tofurkey, soy cheese substitutes, and countless other sources of soy products.

It may be less effective than human estrogen but all those little bits add up when you're using soy and other phytoestrogen-rich plants as your protein source. These may be OK for women, especially anyone going through menopause, but men don't need any extra estrogen. You might see a lot of studies done in the news saying things like "too much soy reduces sperm count" and "overeating of soy products leads to earlier memory loss in men in Indonesia" (Indonesians consume a lot of soy as part of their traditional diet). While the Food and Drug Administration (FDA) hasn't ruled on anything yet, this bad buzz is enough to scare some people away and make others think twice.

Unfortunately, this fact (and the fact that not everyone is going to like tofu no matter who they are) scares people away from even trying the vegetarian diet.

Chia is unique among seeds for many reasons, all of which are beneficial to you! First off, by weight, the chia seed is 23 percent complete protein. The chia seed's protein level makes it a valuable dietary addition for vegetarians.

This tiny seed has other wonderful benefits that can be taken advantage of especially by men. Chia seeds don't have plant estrogens to mess with the hormone balance that keeps you healthy. They don't require you to learn how to cook with tofu (and make it taste good—a real feat!). They don't require lots of preparation time or know-how in the kitchen. You don't have to change your eating habits. Basically, if you have a measuring spoon or scoop, you can use chia—whether you're a vegetarian or not!

Chia seeds are loaded with bonus benefits. Want better regularity? Chia is packed with soluble and insoluble fiber. Insoluble fiber acts as a "sweeper" in the intestine, keeping food moving along. Soluble fiber irrigates the bowels, making digestion easier so that the intestines don't have to work as hard to move food. Enough fiber in your diet also helps reduce the risk of colon cancer, which studies have shown is more common in men than it is in women.

If you are already a vegetarian, all the anti-soy hype in the news won't bother you when you have chia seeds in the house.

Whatever conclusion the scientific studies come to with regard to plant estrogens, you'll know you're safe with chia seeds.

WHY GO MEATLESS ONE NIGHT PER WEEK?

Have you considered having a meat-free night one day each week? Having one meatless dinner per week can have all kinds of benefits for you and your family. But how can cutting something *out* give you *more*? When you try a meatless night, you'll soon discover benefits like improved nutrition, lower fat, lower costs, and you'll even improve the environment.

One day out of each week isn't much. You don't have to make drastic changes or stop eating the foods you love. With the abundance of delicious recipes, veggie-friendly restaurants, and even meat-free readymade meals available today, it's easy to find something meat-free to choose just one night of the week. This little change is so simple that anyone can do it, and so important that everyone can make a difference.

How much difference can only one night each week make? The climate expert Rajendra Pachauri says that livestock are responsible for 18 percent of the world's greenhouse gas emissions.[25] Eighteen percent might not seem like much, but scientists at the University of Chicago say that if everyone in the United States had *one* meat-free night each week, it would mean the energy equivalent of twelve billion fewer gallons of gasoline each year. Now *that's* a lot saved! But what is it like on a more personal scale? For every 2.2 pounds of beef not consumed, you remove as much carbon dioxide from the air as *not* driving a car 155 miles.

Without all the land cleared for farming animal food, without all the fossil fuel spent on transporting animals and meat around,

---

25   Rajendra Pachauri, "UN Urges Global Move To Meat And Dairy Free Diet," *The Guardian*, http://www.theguardian.com/environment/2010/jun/02/un-report-meat-free-diet (Accessed 18 October 2013)

and without all the animal waste products harming the environment, you already know that cutting out a little meat is good for the planet. But what about you and your family? How can a meat-free night improve your health?

Plant-based foods are naturally low-fat, low in (or free from!) cholesterol, high in vitamins, rich in minerals, and full of healthy fiber. Fiber not only helps you feel full faster but aids in healthy digestion as well. Growth hormones and antibiotics aren't used on plants and most can be cleaned quite well with a safe baking soda wash. High-fiber diets help lower the risk of colon cancer and diverticulitis. Many useful minerals such as iron, calcium, and zinc (usually thought of in milk and meat), are also found in abundance in certain leaves, seeds, and nuts. Chia seeds actually have more calcium by weight than milk and spinach is rich in iron. Some of the longest-lived people on earth eat at least seven servings of vegetables each day (while the USDA recommends only five) and very little meat. Studies have repeatedly shown that a high-vegetable but low-meat diet is very beneficial. Notice that we didn't mention cutting out *all* meat, just lowering your consumption of it! Eating some meat can still be good for you.

By going meat-free one night per week, you can save money. Meat has to be prepared and that's always going to require electricity, whether it's the stove, microwave, or the oven. If you're buying precooked, presliced meats, you can expect to pay more too. The more steps that go into preparing a product, the higher its price will be when it's on the shelf or at the deli.

Now that you know the benefits of adding a meatless night to your schedule, what steps can you take to actually enjoy it? There are plenty of recipes where you won't miss the meat and that don't require tofu or other meat substitutes. If you're worried about not feeling full or not getting enough complete protein from the meal, why not add beans or chia seeds to it? Chia also has calcium, iron, magnesium, and healthy omega-3 oil (which is usually found in fish).

Because it's only one night each week, experimentation is easy. The Internet has made it faster than ever to locate recipes to try. There are many tasty dishes to try with beans. Beans contain a plant protein, fiber, and trace minerals. Many beans are also rich in antioxidants (the darker the bean, the more antioxidants it is likely to provide). Their two kinds of fiber aid with digestion and help fill you up, so it's totally possible to have a hearty meal that contains no meat.

It's up to you to have the fun of discovering great meat free recipes. Recipes of all types are so easy to find with a simple search and you never know what you might discover. Maybe you'll even find your family's new favorite meal!

Want to get started with meatless night right away? Here are some great recipes with fantastic flavors so that you won't even miss the meat!

SWEET POTATO VEGGIE BURGER WITH APPLE GUACAMOLE

You can make this crispy, tasty burger so quickly that you will surprise yourself! As it is a veggie burger, you must either cook your patties on an indoor flat grill or broil them in the oven. These burgers hold together nicely and are packed with awesome flavor and veggie goodness. You may even want to have these even if it's not meatless Monday. Everyone has different heat tolerances, and we are not heat seekers. If you would like to add a little more jalapeño, go ahead, but remember that the heat grows on your palate and you don't want to overshadow other great flavors. The awesome guacamole has just a little zip but does not overpower the burger. It's unconventional and is a bit crunchy, which makes for a wonderful change of pace.

This recipe makes four patties.

INGREDIENTS:

FOR THE PATTIES:

1 small, raw sweet potato (peeled and shredded to equal about 1 cup, packed)

¾ of a 15-oz can of black beans (rinsed)

1 garlic clove (minced)

2 tablespoons red onion (minced)

A sliver of jalapeño, minced (about an eighth of the pepper) or ⅛ teaspoon chili powder

1 teaspoon ground cumin

1 egg

2 tablespoons dry bread crumbs

1 tablespoon dry chia

FOR THE GUACAMOLE:

1 Haas avocado

Small handful of cilantro (de-stemmed and lightly chopped)

2 teaspoons lemon juice

1 teaspoon lime juice

1 garlic clove (minced)

1 tablespoon red onion (minced)

1 jalapeño sliver (minced)

½ green apple (finely chopped)

1 teaspoon dry chia

⅓ cup low-fat sour cream

INSTRUCTIONS:

FOR THE PATTIES:

In a bowl, smash the black bean with a fork. Add the grated sweet potato and the rest of the ingredients. Mix by hand and form into four equal sized balls. Flatten to about one-half inch deep. Coat your grill or cookie sheet with cooking spray. Grill for about four minutes if using closed-top grill such as a George Foreman.

If you will be broiling, cook for about eight minutes and then flip to crisp the other side for about two to three minutes. Or, lightly oil a skillet and cook for three to four minutes, then flip and crisp for another three minutes.

FOR THE GUACAMOLE:

In a small bowl, smash the avocado and add the remaining ingredients. Stir to combine. It would be wise to make your guac first so that the flavors have a change to blend. So, you could then cover and chill it while you put together your patties.

PORTOBELLO MUSHROOM SANDWICH

Mushrooms provide a hearty, meaty texture to sandwiches and other dishes without adding any actual meat. Mushrooms are also extremely nutritious and packed with protein, thiamin, vitamin B6, folate, magnesium, zinc, and manganese. That's not all, though! They are a very good source of dietary fiber, riboflavin, niacin, pantothenic acid, phosphorus, potassium, copper, and selenium.

Do you grill your mushrooms? It just takes about ten minutes in a zip-top sandwich bag with the marinade to have your portobellos ready for either your inside or outside grill. This sandwich has a great flavor with almost a meatiness to it. With a roasted red pepper on top, you will look forward to meatless Mondays when you make these super sandwiches.

INGREDIENTS:

    1 zip-top baggie
    2 portobello caps
    3 tablespoons balsamic vinegar
    1 tablespoon olive oil
    2 cloves of garlic, minced
    2 large strips roasted red pepper

A sprinkle of chia seeds (to stick to the pepper before placing on the sandwich)
  Bread or bun of your choice
  Baby arugula (optional)
  Red onion (optional)

INSTRUCTIONS:

Simply add the mushrooms, vinegar, oil, and minced garlic to the baggie and zip it! Marinade for at least ten minutes and you are ready to grill indoors or out doors for about ten minutes, turning once. Toast the bread if desired. Place the mushroom on your bread base and top the mushroom with a roasted red pepper strip and the chia seeds, add the lid and prepare to enjoy. These sandwiches work really well with the chia side dishes found in this book (e.g., the avocado soup that follows). Make it a chia meal!

CREAMY AVOCADO CHIA SOUP

This soup is cool, light, and refreshing and is paired up with so many garden goodies! The "creamy" comes from low-fat plain yogurt with just a little Greek yogurt to give it a zing. Don't warm this soup as we certainly don't want to kill all the good yogurt bacteria that keep our bodies in balance. Choose a probiotic yogurt for maximum health benefits! Fast and easy to prepare, this is our go-to soup when avocados are in season.

INGREDIENTS:

  2 ripe Haas avocados
  1 lemon (juiced, about 2 tablespoons)
  1 cup low-fat plain yogurt
  ½ cup Greek yogurt
  2 cups vegetable stock (low sodium is best)

2 small carrots
2 large basil leaves (slivered)
2 tablespoons chia gel
⅛ teaspoon cayenne pepper

Garnish options: black beans, diced tomato, diced carrot, a few kernels of corn, diced cucumber, parsley, sliced radishes, torn fresh spinach . . . whatever is in your fridge!

INSTRUCTIONS:

This is *so* easy and requires almost zero kitchen utensils. Place the avocado flesh in a large, flat-bottomed bowl or casserole dish. Smash with a fork but leave some small chunks so that the soup has a great texture. Stir in the yogurts and the veggie stock.

With a grater or vegetable peeler, cut long strands of carrot to make "noodles." The carrot strands should be no longer than an inch or two so that eating the soup is not difficult. Add the carrot "noodles," slivered basil leaves, lemon juice, chia gel, and cayenne pepper. Let the soup rest so that the flavors can blend. Chill if serving later.

Chia Seeds versus Various Maladies

Chia seeds can be used to help with a variety of conditions. Most of these conditions are brought on by commonly available food choices (e.g., processed foods without much fiber). In this section, you can learn how chia seeds can be used in different ways to help bring relief or eliminate certain dietary-related problems. By using nutrition to power up your immune system, you can also avoid many maladies as well. Your immune system is your first line of defense against so many problems. You can also learn how to avoid cumulative damage from inflammation to enjoy good health for much longer.

Do you want the ultimate disease fighting weapon? It can take on viruses and bacteria no matter how many times they mutate. This amazing weapon even fights off mutant cells, foreign items, and cancer cells. The real fact is that you already have this weapon at your disposal right now, and it is your own immune system. Your immune system is made of multiple parts and is highly complex and sophisticated. It's also your best line of defense against threats such as viruses and bacteria that would otherwise destroy your cells. It battles many intruders every day as you go about your normal routine. You don't even notice as it fights off threats to your health—that's just how powerful it is.

With health scares like the bird flu, the swine flu (H1N1), and flu season in general, plus antibiotic-resistant bacteria surfacing each year, it's important now more than ever to be protected. No one else is able to defend you from disease, so it's important that *you* take every action you can to stay safe this season, and every season.

First, take safe actions. Washing your hands frequently (the soap doesn't even have to be antibacterial; remember, viruses are different than bacteria—but either one will slide off when you use soap), especially before you eat, prepare food, apply makeup, or use your toothbrush. Other safe actions include *never* covering your mouth and nose with your hand when you sneeze or cough, *always* use your elbow instead. Germs are spread most easily through other people touching them, and then touching their face or their food. Your elbow rarely touches other surfaces throughout your day. Getting enough sleep is also a safe action because when your body has enough rest, it is better able to fend off problems.

Second, power up your immune system. Like all parts of the body, your immune system needs fuel to run on. There are several easy ways to help boost your immunity and none of them are expensive or dangerous. Have you heard negative reports about flu vaccination preservatives, for example, that they could contain too much mercury? (Mercury is a toxic heavy metal but it is sometimes used as a preservative agent in vaccines.) Whether you get vaccinated every year (for flu season, etc.) or not, your immune system needs to be in top shape. If you think vaccines like the one for swine flu (H1N1) aren't safe to take or you're just worried about the negative press their preservative agents get, it is especially important to protect yourself in other ways.

The first way is by supplementing with vitamins. Vitamin C is the most popular immunity booster, and even though it's found in foods you may like such as oranges, kiwis, and other citrus fruits, it's still a good idea to supplement with it to ensure you get at least 1,000 milligrams per day. Vitamin C is water soluble, so it is hard to get too much of it. Vitamin D is another big immunity booster. Your body can make it if you're exposed to fifteen minutes of sunlight each day, but what if the sun is weak, it is cloudy, or you just can't find the time to be outside? It's simple and cheap to use vitamin D3 pills. These pills are tiny, about the size of a piece of corn, and are so inexpensive that it can be under $0.05 per day to use them. The research on vitamin D is so important that Canada is even recommending it to the population to help prevent against swine flu.

Third, increase your overall health. When your body is in good shape, your immune system isn't distracted by preexisting problems. The best ways to increase your health include getting enough sleep each night, avoiding as much stress as possible, and consuming a diet of healthy foods. Eating maximum health foods such as fruits, vegetables, nuts, seeds, and lean, free-range meat can really help you out. Not only do they give you more energy for your day, they also provide the nutrients your immune system needs to help keep you safe. These nutrients also include trace minerals (items you only need a tiny amount of, but are important nonetheless!). Trace minerals include selenium, boron, magnesium, copper, and zinc. Leafy greens, vegetables, and fruits get these from the soil and deliver them to you.

Want to boost the nutrition of the foods you already like to eat? No matter how healthy some foods are, you don't want to eat them at every meal. Broccoli for breakfast? Bell peppers for dessert? No one wants that. But what if you could boost the nutrition of foods you already like to eat? You could add calcium and boron to your oatmeal, yogurt, or cereal for breakfast. You could add healthy omega-3 oil (usually found in fish) to your sandwich at lunch, without ever touching a fish. You could even add the same protein found in meats to non-meat dishes. Just add chia! Being able to boost the nutrition of foods you already like makes it easy enough that anyone can have better immune health.

When you take safe actions and boost your immune system with healthy foods and vitamins, you're much less likely to get sick. No matter how scary the news makes the latest health threat out to be, your immune system is your best defense. Keep it in top shape and you'll feel better year-round!

CHIA HELPS PREVENT DIVERTICULITIS

Diverticulitis seems to be the new "disease of the year" in the media. Everywhere you turn you're hearing more doctors and medical studies say, "More people in the world have either diverticulitis or diverticulosis than ever before!" But how many of them are telling you effective and easy ways you may be able to use to stop it? Certainly not many.

It's time for a change, and it's time for *you* to take control of your digestive health. However, for you to be fully in charge, you need to understand the facts. When you're armed with what's really going on, it makes it so much easier to reveal the easy changes you can make to prevent this painful problem.

First, these intestinal changes don't develop overnight. Because of dietary habits, the problem takes a while to form and then be noticed by the affected person. *Diverticulum* are small pockets in the intestine wall that develop when the intestine has to work too hard to move food through it. The great strain causes these hazardous pockets to form. They can become infected and sore or even break open and harm your health.

But why do they form? And why now more than ever? It's not your fault! Just look around at the foods readily available to everyone. They're full of refined flour and there isn't a lot of whole grain that tastes delicious as an option for you. The combination of not enough liquid throughout the day plus not enough soluble and insoluble fiber adds up to intestinal trouble.

Fiber is important for your health on many different levels. Once you understand the benefits of fiber, you can use it to combat many common problems! There are five main points to keep in mind.

First, fiber that is incompletely or slowly digested promotes normal bowel function and treats constipation. This type of fiber also helps prevent diverticulosis and diverticulitis. It provides relief from irritable bowel syndrome (IBS), which is also on the rise.

Second, fiber-rich foods are processed more slowly by the body. This is a great benefit if you're trying to lose weight! When foods process more slowly, you feel satisfied or full much faster than normal. This makes it easy to eat less at mealtime.

Third, by packing in fiber, the food you eat is less calorically dense. The fiber fills you up and performs its important roles, but it *isn't* absorbed by the body to turn into extra calories and fat. Certain kinds of fiber can never be digested; they're sometimes called *roughage*.

Fourth, reduce your risk of colon cancer. When the food you eat has enough fiber in it, it does not spend very long in the intestines. Bile acid doesn't get reabsorbed. Unwelcome bacteria don't get a chance to ferment food in the intestines. Toxins don't build up or have the opportunity to be absorbed into the body because everything keeps on moving. Thirteen case-control studies were recently published on the use of fiber in the diet.[26] They concluded with substantiated evidence that the risk of colorectal cancer in the United States could be decreased by 31 percent *just* by adding thirteen grams more fiber each day. Easy to do? Just keep reading.

Fifth, fiber can help with cholesterol and blood glucose. Everyone knows about cholesterol levels, good and bad. There have been so many studies on this as a risk factor for heart attacks and heart disease. There's plenty you can do naturally to help lower cholesterol, but did you know that getting enough fiber will help too? Soluble fiber has been proven to lower blood cholesterol levels.

But what about glucose? Glucose and insulin levels are important for preventing type-2 diabetes. Starchy foods, sugary drinks, and other modern day diet options that convert quickly into sugars in the body spike insulin levels. These are hard on your body to digest, so you can give your system a break with fiber. Viscous fiber (which appears like a gelatin) slows down the conversion of carbohydrates into sugars and helps normalize blood glucose levels.

But if fiber is so beneficial, why isn't anyone getting enough? There's plenty of fiber in apple peels, celery stalks, whole grains such as oat and flax but these foods don't always fit into what people think is delicious or convenient. "An apple a day . . ." is rarely practiced by anyone! What about fiber pills or powders? These can be expensive, gritty, or "just another pill" among a handful that people already don't really want to choke down every day. Plus, with supplement pills or powders, the body misses out on important oils, micronutrients, and antioxidants available in plant fiber sources.

---

26   WebMD.com, "High Fiber Diet Linked to Lower Colon Cancer Risk," http://www.webmd.com/colorectal-cancer/news/20111110/high-fiber-diet-linked-to-lower-colon-cancer-risk (Accessed 18 October 2013)

What can *you* do about it? The power to save yourself from this range of digestive maladies is now in your hands. Now that you have a basic understanding of what fiber can do for you and how it works, it's time to take easy action and start using chia seeds. When you're adding chia gel to drinks or sprinkling chia onto foods you already like, you're adding fiber without losing flavor. Even low fiber foods like a white-bread bagel can be made to have a portion of your daily fiber intake when you sprinkle chia seeds onto it. Be sure to read about probiotics and prebiotics, the handy section in this book; there are even more great benefits to fiber than you'd think!

There are plenty of recipes out there that feature fiber-rich foods. Fiber doesn't have to be bland, boring, gritty, or a chore. Get started with these cool fiber rich recipes.

INTRODUCING FIBER

Studies have shown that people who eat plenty of fiber have healthy colons teeming with bacteria. Science has shown us that gut flora on fiber creates an acidic environment in the colon so that the risk of developing diverticulitis or colorectal cancer is at a minimum. We often use Greek yogurt in our recipes instead of high-calorie, high-fat mayonnaise because of the live and active bacterial cultures. These cultures are especially important to replace if you have just finished an antibiotic treatment. The antibiotic kills all the good and bad "bugs" in your stomach.

Just by keeping your "plumbing" unclogged, you could lower your risk of colon cancer as much as 43 percent, according to a recent British study.[27]

How much fiber should you have? According to the latest government guidelines, your total fiber intake should be about

---

27 Cancer Research uk.org, "UK Diet and Cancer: The Evidence," http://www.cancerresearchuk.org/cancer-info/healthyliving/dietandhealthyeating/howdoweknow/ (Accessed 22 October 2013)

twenty grams to forty grams daily. Most people in the United States are ingesting less than twenty grams per day. Yikes! The government guideline may even be low. A breakfast cereal that proclaims "a good source of fiber" may only have three grams of fiber. Sprinkling, stirring in, or adding chia to your new lifestyle will help you get more of the fiber you need. It's easy!

If you're eating dry chia seeds or sprinkling a lot of dry chia onto your favorite foods to add fiber, remember to drink plenty of water. This goes for any type of high-fiber food as well, not just chia. If you don't drink enough water with your fiber, you can get stomach cramps. Fiber tends to absorb liquids. If you add dry fiber to your stomach, it can absorb any or all of the liquid in the stomach which can cause it to give you a cramping sensation. So remember to have a nice, healthy drink on hand with every snack and meal.

The soluble fiber on the outside of the chia seed shell really helps out your intestines!

Because the soluble fibers are very good at holding onto water, that liquid isn't easy for the body to remove. Chia seeds may stay hydrated all the way through to the large intestine. This is great news because the more moisture that's retained to this point in digestion, the better off the colon is. When the large intestine has lots of really moist food and ready access to water, it can function at its best. There's no struggling to move food and nothing harmful has the chance to linger in the body.

The American Dietetic Association has also released that soluble fiber helps lower serum cholesterol. Not only is soluble fiber a cholesterol buster, scientists believe that eating a fiber-rich diet may help reduce diabetes and heart disease too. Fiber is good for so much more than just intestinal health.

Have you heard of bile acid? Bile acid is a byproduct of digestion. It helps break down fats in foods, but it's not something you want to absorb. Normally, bile acid is used then sequestered and passed out of the body so that it doesn't get absorbed by the intestine. Because cholesterol is used to create bile acid, the body will use up part of its cholesterol supply to manufacture more. That's good news for you, because that action lowers cholesterol levels by putting the cholesterol molecules to good use.

The intestines' job is to absorb nutrients and transfer them properly into the bloodstream. However, if something unhealthy is present in the intestine for a long period of time, it can be accidentally absorbed. Improperly digested food can smother good bacteria and allow bad bacteria to ferment and create excess gas. Bile acid can rise to higher-than-normal levels on a high-fat diet. Because bile acid is used to break down fats, when a high-fat diet is consumed, naturally the liver will produce lots of bile acid to help break down those fats. Bile acid becomes a problem when a high-fat but low-fiber diet is consumed. You want to use up bile acid; it has to do its job, and then exit the body. However, when there's not enough fiber in the colon along with the fats, the food and the fats and the bile acid and the bad bacteria all linger around and have a chance at getting absorbed, which can harm your health. Studies have shown that colon cancer can even be a result of improperly digested food, bad bacteria, and various byproducts lingering in the intestines.

How should you introduce more fiber into your meal plans? As you plan to increase your fiber, do it gradually to give your body time to adjust to your new lifestyle. Drink plenty of water to balance the quantity of water the fiber will absorb in your gut. Some people just load up on fiber, have digestive consequences, and then simply say, "Well, fiber doesn't work for me." If constipation is a problem for you, your body is speaking loudly to you but you are not listening! Remember that alcohol, caffeine, and artificial sweeteners can be a diuretic. The liquid these beverages provide can be dismissed too quickly by the body. If the kidneys are filtering and flushing out caffeinated liquid quickly, the water portion of the drink never gets to the intestine to be used for irrigation of the fiber you ate.

A healthy bowel has an ideal balance of good and bad bacteria. Doctors recommend about 80 percent good and 20 percent bad. (There's no way to get rid of all the bad bacteria, you just need the good guys to outnumber them significantly.) This is just about the opposite of what most people contain in their gut. The bowel's contents need to move with an adequate supply of fiber and water. A bacterial imbalance can lead to many maladies, such as irritable bowel symptoms, acid reflux, gum disease, painful joints, yeast problems, food sensitivities, fatigue, and malnutrition.

Exercise helps keeps your bowels moving as well as you. If you realize you're not getting enough fiber and you want to introduce more fiber into your diet, consider adding exercise as well. You've read how exercise helps reduce stress, lets you sleep better, and makes you feel more fit. Set a few short-term goals for yourself. Once you get into the routine you probably will start looking forward to it, and you can impress yourself!

If you feel bloated or have excessive gas, eat slowly and chew thoroughly, as you will swallow less air. You may want to avoid some of the more "gassy" foods such as carbonated drinks, beans, and artificial sweeteners, such as anything with "itol" at the end of the word, for a while. (The artificial sweeteners with the "itol" suffix—yes, this does include xylitol, the natural one of the bunch—have been known to create excess gas as a side effect in some people.)

Some people don't have the type and or quantity of bacteria or enzymes to digest beans and certain other high-fiber veggies. When these high-fiber foods aren't digested properly, they form a sludge, which is delivered to the large intestine almost intact. That is where the fermentation and bloating may occur. By the time food reaches the colon, it's supposed to be very broken down and basic.

If you are sensitive to beans or cruciferous veggies, you could take an enzyme supplement specifically formulated for such foods before eating them until your body adjusts. The benefits of fiber are well worth experimenting with different enzyme product helpers, and it's also worth the general, easy experimentation you may need to do with your menu when you're first introducing more fiber to your meal plan.

Grandma was right, although she didn't know why. The answer is, rinsing your beans in fresh, cool water washes off excess salt from packaging or processing and excess starch too. The starch can leach out of beans when they're cooked and canned. Rinsing it away in a colander can help your beans taste better, and agree with you better as well.

Grandma's second tip: you could try having a teaspoon of apple cider vinegar before dinner. You may notice that many of our bean-incorporated dinners have dressing with apple cider vinegar included. If you have no medical problems, maybe just the slow increase of these veggies and the probiotics found in the plain yogurts may up your healthy bacteria and not cause an embarrassing moment.

The bathroom should not be the library. When you are consuming the "right-for-your-body-with-plenty-of-fiber" foods, and adding plenty of water and some exercise, you won't be able to read a paragraph in your book. Your goal should be easy elimination almost every day.

CHUNKY CHIA TABBOULEH

This is an easy and tasty way to use your leftover lentils. We usually prepare about two cups of lentils and then freeze about half for another use in salads or soups. (What a time saver!) We believe that this gorgeous side salad goes well with just about everything! (Well, maybe not chocolate cake.)

INGREDIENTS:

FOR THE TABBOULEH:

    1 cup of prepared lentils (your color choice)

    2 diced tomatoes

    2 ¼-inch slices of red onion, diced

    1 large cucumber

    1 small carrot

    1 large handful of parsley, stems removed and chopped

FOR THE DRESSING:

    ¼ cup olive oil

    2 tablespoons apple cider vinegar

    2 tablespoons fresh lime juice

    1 tablespoon dry chia seeds

    1 dash black pepper

    ½ tablespoon dried mint

INSTRUCTIONS:

In a large casserole or bowl combine the chopped vegetables with room-temperature cooked lentils. In a small measuring cup combine the dressing ingredients. If you are asking yourself, why didn't we use fresh mint? The answer is that the dried mint flavor permeated the dish so well that we were just happy with this fresh flavor!

CARIBBEAN MANGO CHIA SLAW

You can have a taste of summer all year long with this low-fat and high-flavor coleslaw. Frozen mango can be used if mangos aren't in season, which can make this a go-to side any time of the year. This fast, easy, zippy slaw makes a great side dish to build your meal around. You can even send your burgers on a lovely vacation from the traditional tomato, lettuce, and mayo too when you top them with slaw. It is great to have a little crunch and fresh flavor sitting right under your bun!

INGREDIENTS:

½ a bag of coleslaw mix (about 6 ounces)

1 mango, skinned and chopped into bite-size pieces (or 1 cup of frozen mango chunks, thawed)

1 small sweet red pepper, deseeded and minced

1 small handful of de-stemmed parsley

⅓ cup nonfat plain yogurt

1 teaspoon prepared yellow mustard

1 tablespoon apple cider vinegar

1 teaspoon agave or honey

1 teaspoon chia

1 dash cayenne pepper

INSTRUCTIONS:

In a medium bowl place the coleslaw mix, mango, red pepper, and parsley. In a measuring cup mix the yogurt, mustard, vinegar, and agave. Stir to combine. Add the chia and a dash of cayenne pepper. Stir again and pour the dressing over the slaw mixture and stir to combine.

Note: We love this slaw on a turkey burger. To create a zippy burger, just add a little less than one-half teaspoon of grated ginger and a dash of pepper flakes to the meat before you cook it. A Caribbean ticket for your taste buds!

Also, did you know that cabbage is made up of approximately 92 percent water. Cabbage delivers a good dose of many essential vitamins, including C, K, E, and A, minerals, and dietary fiber, plus folic acid. It is a natural diuretic that can help expel excess fluids from the body. It's packed with glucosinolates, organic compounds that contain nitrogen and sulfur, which help flush out unwanted toxins too.

DISCOVER FIVE WAYS YOU CAN CURB ACID INDIGESTION SAFELY WITH CHIA

Do you suffer from acid indigestion? Are you worried about acid reflux? Many people feel the burn of acid indigestion or heartburn more than one time each week. Of course there are ways to deal with it if you use chalky tablets or take expensive medications. Everyone's body is different and there are different triggers and solutions. Chia is a helper, it's not going to solve every person's acid indigestion problems all of the time.

What is heartburn? *Heartburn* is the upward backflow of the stomach's contents in the esophagus. If left untreated, this acid burn can cause all sorts of problems, even cancer. The National Cancer Institute states, "In the United States, the prevalence of esophageal cancer has increased 850 percent since 1975." Dr. Jamie Koufman, a professor at New York Medical College, mainly blames the acid-ification of the American diet, along with increased saturated fats and high fructose corn syrup (HFC) and agricultural pesticides. Dr. Koufman believes that high-acidic diets and soft drinks are the major risk factor for reflux. Acid reflux really begins in the stomach where the enzyme pepsin breaks down proteins. Your stomach is activated by the acid in the high-acid foods. "If there is no protein around that needs digesting, pepsin can gnaw on the lining of your throat and esophagus," explains Koufman.[28] You can give any meal some protein with chia seeds.

Wouldn't it be great if there was an all-natural and inexpensive solution that actually enriches your diet while relieving you of your acid problems? The solution may be unexpected, but it is exceptional! It's chia seeds to the rescue once again.

To relieve indigestion, all you need to do is eat one dry teaspoon of chia, and drink a few mouthfuls of filtered water. Right away,

28   Jamie Koufman, "Banish Acid Reflux: Eating Alkaline Can Cure The Burn," *Natural Awakenings Magazine*, http://www.naturalawakeningsmag.com/ Natural-Awakenings/July-2013/Banish-Acid-Reflux/ (Accessed 18 October 2013)

the tiny seeds will go to work in your stomach to help you feel better. Some people could need more than one teaspoon. Let your body be your guide; wait ten minutes and see if you feel better—if not, you can add more chia.

Let's take a look at how chia seeds help you fight off heart burn.

First, super-absorbent quality: Each tiny seed is covered in a soluble fiber layer. When the seed is dry, this layer isn't visible to the naked eye. However, when you wet the seed and wait ten minutes, you'll see that a big bead of gel (with the consistency of a gelatin snack) has formed around the seed. This shows that the soluble fiber has been activated. The tiny fibers grab and hold onto liquid, keeping it on the surface of the seed.

How it helps you: This absorbent quality isn't limited to water. The seeds will soak up almost any liquid they're added to, including stomach irritants. They'll form the beads of gel and be passed through into the intestines, which then safely remove the gels and release the nutrients in the seed.

Second, clinging quality: In the process of forming gels, the seeds may also gather up impurities in the liquid. The ancient Aztec people, if they got dirt or ash in their eyes in battle, would actually allow a chia seed to be dropped into the eye. (This is not recommended; you are not an ancient Aztec warrior.) The seed would then go to work absorbing their eye's water and any debris along with it. The seed and debris could then be easily removed, and the eye was clear again.

The same thing happens when dry seeds are added to your stomach. Particles, bacteria, and liquids are captured when the seeds form their gel.

Third, alkaline quality: Chia seeds aren't acidic. They won't add to your problem; their alkaline quality will help balance you out. Chia contains six times more calcium than whole milk (by weight), which is not only good for your bones but also good for your digestive health. Chia seeds also include the trace mineral boron, which is an important key for absorbing calcium.

Fourth, double-fiber quality: Chia contains more fiber than flax seeds and bran flakes. It provides both soluble and insoluble fiber, both of which are necessary for healthy digestion. Fiber helps move food through the digestive tract. Not only does this prevent constipation, it sweeps out substances that may be harming you, such as bacteria waste and bile acid. When everything is moving along quickly, toxic wastes don't get the chance to build up in your intestines. When your digestion is right on track, acid reflux is less likely to occur in the future.

Fifth, carb-conversion slowdown: When you eat chia seeds, they slow down the conversion of carbohydrates into sugars. This not only has the benefit of helping to balance blood sugar, it also helps you feel satisfied sooner. Traditional advice for acid indigestion avoidance usually includes "stay away from sweets" because a sugar overload could trigger an acid incident. When you use chia, you can help avoid a sweet overload.

Chia seeds are 100 percent safe and natural. Pesticides and GMOs aren't used in growing them. They are free of any chemicals or additives. Because of these amazing properties, they never need enhancement of any kind. You don't have to be afraid of any sort of overdose when you use them. You can eat chia every day, forever, and you'll only become healthier because of it!

The same can't be said for PPIs or H2 antagonists (also called acid blockers). These are a type of pharmaceutical drug that inhibits the body's ability to produce acid. They work very well, even in over-the-counter form. However, if used for any longer than the recommended amount of time by either the label or your doctor, they can create real trouble for you.

Antacids and acid blocker problems: When used for extended periods against product recommendations, these drugs prevent your body from absorbing calcium and B12. This reduces bone density and can even lead to osteoporosis. The level of people afflicted with osteoporosis is on the rise in America, especially in men. This quote from a professional pharmacist, Jim LaValle, RPh, ND, CCN, states the problem: "Recently, I did some radio and TV interviews on the topic of osteoporosis. Rates are increasing, especially in men; 55 percent of people over the age fifty have osteoporosis and another thirty-four million or so have low bone density. As a pharmacist, I feel obligated to warn people that one of the contributing factors to these increased rates is taking prescription and over-the-counter drugs that reduce or block the production of gastric acid. I'm talking about proton pump inhibitors (PPIs) and other acid-blocking drugs like H2 antagonists for heartburn and ulcers. Besides lowering B12 absorption, which influences red blood cells and homocysteine levels, these drugs reduce stomach acid so effectively that they keep your body from absorbing calcium, and therefore can reduce bone density."[29]

You don't have to live with acid indigestion or sacrifice your bone health. With chia on hand, you can combat acid safely and healthfully when it acts up. It doesn't block the production of acid, which you need to absorb vital minerals. It actually provides you with calcium and the full range of B vitamins, not to mention complete protein and fiber. It's also inexpensive, costing less than $1 per day, even if you use it several times a day. When you use chia, maintain a smart and healthy diet, and don't overload on caffeine and alcohol, you may be looking at the end of costly and painful digestive problems. Chia can only help you, so why not give it a try today?

---

29   Jim LaValle, R.Ph, ND, CCN, "Why Osteoporosis is On The Rise," *X1 Concepts* http://www.x1concept.com/blog/tag/osteoporosis/ (Accessed 18 October 2013)

A LITTLE BIT ABOUT DIGESTION

Knowing how something works can help you understand the process better or make changes to help fix something that's gone wrong. With sections such as "Alkaline versus Acidic Diets" and tips on fighting acidosis, you might think that we're against acid but that's just not true! Stomach acid is very important for your health, and it's actually one of the first lines of defense for the immune system. Before we can even talk about stomach acid, we need to spend a little time talking about how it fits in the digestive process. Acid is meant to be a helper, killing bad bacteria and viruses and breaking down food. Many people believe that only acid can break down food. Because acid is only one component of digestion, it can't work all by itself, and that's where problems come in.

Did you know that digestion actually starts in the mouth? Saliva has enzymes that begin breaking down food as soon as you start chewing. Enzymes in the mouth are different from ones in the stomach and small intestine. Enzymes are like a team of tiny keys, each one unlocking different nutrients from your food. To get the best out of all the nutrients, you need a variety of these tiny keys.

Be sure to chew your food thoroughly! Lots of chewing produces lots of saliva to get the enzymes started on your meal. People who eat in a rush, people who eat lots of very soft foods, and people who aren't paying any attention to how they are eating (i.e., distracted eating, such as while driving, watching TV, or playing video games) can eat too quickly and fail to chew enough to properly start up digestion. This can lead to heartburn later on.

Ideally, with enough chewing the food would enter the stomach laced with digestive enzymes. These enzymes would then "predigest" your food for about an hour, still inside the stomach—actually breaking down as much as 75 percent of your meal. (That's a big job for just a little saliva!)

Only after this period of pre-digestion are hydrochloric acid and pepsin released into the stomach. Stomach acid inactivates all of the food-based and saliva-based enzymes. (Foods such as papaya are known for their healthy enzyme content—it's a food that helps you break it down!) Now the acid begins breaking down what is left of the meal in combination with the acid-energized enzyme pepsin. Pepsin is one of the few enzymes that can actually function in the harsh environment of an acid-filled stomach. When the food leaves the stomach and enters the small intestine, the acid is neutralized and the pancreas is then able to reintroduce digestive enzymes to the process safely. As digestion is completed, nutrients are passed through the intestinal wall and into the bloodstream.

Processing and cooking destroys enzymes in food. Enzymes are not alive but they can be deactivated or destroyed. Freezing will deactivate only a very few; they're fairly resistant to freezing. However, heating anywhere above 180 degrees Fahrenheit will deactivate most enzymes in most foods. Remember that all bottled juices and all canned goods have been heated above 180 degrees in their packing process. To ensure you're getting enough enzymes, fix fresh foods for yourself.

Without enzymes and without enough chewing, the food enters the stomach in an "unprepared state." This forces the body to produce large amounts of stomach acid in an attempt to overcompensate. The stomach has to attempt to make up for what the enzymes couldn't break down. This excess acid can contribute to acid reflux and heartburn. You might also try an enzyme supplement with a meal. If you know that the food you want to eat isn't enzyme-rich or has been cooked at more than 180 degrees Fahrenheit (like lasagna, for example), an enzyme supplement could help you avoid the burn later, without hindering your digestion.

Now that you know more about how digestion works, you can help yourself or a friend or family member take a closer look at what causes the heartburn sensation, rather than just attempting to treat the symptoms of heartburn. Chewing food thoroughly, eating enzyme rich foods that have not been deactivated through heat, not eating too quickly, and eating more natural fibrous foods are all unconventional ways to fight acid indigestion.

CHIA SEEDS FOR DIABETES

If you've noticed the news, type-2 diabetes is on the rise in the United States and around the world for both kids and adults. If you don't have it, it's not too late to take steps to prevent it. And if you already have it, there's a way to help manage it. Studies have proven that the earlier you tackle any blood sugar problems, the better your chances are for success.[30] It has also been made clear that losing excess weight can help ward off diabetes. If you could lose weight without being hungry and if you could eat something that tasted however you wanted it to, would you do it?

Get ready for a double shot of weight-loss benefits.

First, chia seeds help you feel full longer and you can actually watch the process work! Diet pills may ask you to believe they work, but chia shows you. If you take one tablespoonful of chia and add it to nine tablespoons of water, stir, and wait fifteen minutes, you'll see that each seed has formed a big bead of gel on the surface and the water is now thick like a gelatin. Notice how much larger this solid form is? This is what happens when you eat the seeds. The gel won't come off the seed easily and is made of pure water. This feels like food in the stomach but replaces calories with water (which has zero calories).

Second, chia is a fiber-rich seed. It has soluble and insoluble fiber. In fact, you can literally *see* the fiber of the chia seed in action

---

30 Associated Press, "Diabetic's Early Blood Sugar Control Can Lower Risks Later," *USA Today*, http://usatoday30.usatoday.com/news/health/2008–09–10-diabetes-control_N.htm (Accessed 22 October 2013)

if you place it in liquid (it will form a big bead of gel around the seed). Fiber-rich foods are processed more slowly by the body. This is a great benefit if you're trying to lose weight without starving! When foods process more slowly, you feel satisfied or full much faster than normal. This makes it easy to eat less at mealtime.

By packing in fiber, the food you eat is less calorically dense. The fiber fills you up and performs its important roles in the colon but *isn't* absorbed by the body to turn into extra calories and fat. Insoluble fiber is not digested. It is sometimes called *roughage* and helps clean the colon.

Blood sugar naturally rises and falls throughout the day. It can also be what makes you drowsy in the afternoon. Dips and spikes aren't good for consistent, healthy energy. The slowing of the conversion of carbohydrates into sugar has the ability to create endurance. Carbohydrates are the fuel for energy in the body. Prolonging their conversion into sugar stabilizes metabolic changes, diminishing the surges of highs and lows, creating a longer duration in their fueling effects. Protein fuels energy as well, and the protein in chia is complete—once again, a double benefit for you.

With chia seeds you can deal a powerful one-two punch against type-2 diabetes risk factors: excess weight and insulin-spiking foods. Of course, there are many other benefits to chia as well, such as healthy omega-3 oils, micronutrients, a full range of B vitamins, and more calcium by weight than milk. If you already have type-2 diabetes, it's important to watch your blood sugar closely and ask your doctor about adding chia seeds to your diet. If you don't have this problem, it's not too late to stop it from ever hitting you. If you have risk factors or if you're just looking for a way to feel better every day and improve your health, you need to take action right away. You need chia seeds!

Here are some recipes that use ingredients that are low on the glycemic index. Low-carb doesn't have to mean low-flavor when you try these recipes with chia. The sweetener here is stevia.

Did you know that stevia has been revealed by a Japanese study to help prevent cavities, strengthen bones, and increase bone-mineral density?[31] This zero–glycemic index sweetener can be a great choice for your recipes.

CHIA GARLICKY CHICKEN VEGGIE STIR-FRY

When you need a fast meal with low carbs and no sugar (we use the stevia leaf, and stevia products are a natural sugar substitute), nothing beats a stir-fry. The slow and steady processing of carbohydrates and the great flavors of this meal makes watching your blood sugar easy and tasty. The chia gel slows down conversion of carbs and blends the flavors too!

INGREDIENTS:

For the sauce:

½ cup chicken or vegetable broth

2 tablespoons low sodium soy sauce

1 teaspoon stevia powder (or your choice of sugar substitute, to equal 1 tablespoon sugar)

1 ½ tablespoons cornstarch

1 tablespoon dry chia

For the rest of the stir-fry:

1 chicken breast, cut into bite-sized strips

5 cloves garlic, minced

3 thin slices of red onion, minced

1 teaspoon fresh ginger, grated

1 to 2 tablespoons olive oil

---

31   Jami Cooley, RN CNWC, "Stevia Benefits Bone Health And More" Article Part Two, *Natural Health Advisory Daily*, http://www.naturalhealthadvisory.com/daily/osteoporosis-prevention-and-treatment/natural-sugar-substitute-stevia-benefits-bone-health-and-more/ (Accessed 18 October 2013)

1 small red pepper, thinly sliced
1 cup broccoli florets
1 cup zucchini, cut into chunks
A handful of fresh mushrooms, sliced
A handful of cabbage slaw
½ cup vegetable broth or chicken broth

INSTRUCTIONS:

In a small measuring cup, first stir together the sauce so that the chia has time to hydrate and set the cup aside.

Second, prepare all the veggies and the chicken bites so that you are ready to quickly cook this speedy supper.

Heat your wok or skillet for thirty seconds, then swirl in one tablespoon of oil and wait for about twenty seconds. Quickly stir-fry the minced garlic, ginger, and diced onion for about sixty seconds. Add the chicken strips and stir-fry until no longer pink inside, about two to three minutes. Add all the vegetables to the wok with the remaining half-cup of broth and cover to steam for a minute or two, so that veggies will be crisp-tender. Remove the lid and add the sauce to coat the ingredients. Continue stirring over the heat until the sauce thickens. Serve immediately.

Note: Some people like a few red pepper flakes added for a little heat. Those who are not watching their carbohydrates as closely as people with diabetes may want to serve this over brown rice. Tailor this recipe with the veggies you like and know you can eat while still keeping your sugar numbers in line. Notice that we have not included corn as corn is a grain, not a vegetable, and it is loaded with sugar!

TOMATO BASIL DRESSING

Tomato lovers unite! This tangy dressing dresses your salad with tomato, tomato, tomato flavor. With no sugars and no fats, it is a diabetic dream come true. Are you tired of having the "same ol' salads"? Change it up a bit with this easy dressing. Leave time to let the chia do its work to blend the flavors in the fridge for about fifteen minutes. This recipe makes about one-half cup of dressing.

INGREDIENTS:
⅓ cup all-natural roasted garlic tomato sauce
¼ cup low-fat plain yogurt
½ teaspoon Worcestershire sauce
1 tablespoon apple cider vinegar
½ teaspoon dried basil
¼ teaspoon tarragon
½ teaspoon dry chia

INSTRUCTIONS;
Use your favorite brand of roasted garlic tomato sauce. Most brands come in about four-ounce cans. Place all the ingredients into a small container with a lid. Do your preliminary taste test and adjust to your liking, bearing in mind that the flavors have not blended yet. Stir to combine. Put on the lid and refrigerate for about fifteen minutes so that the chia seeds will blend the flavors together. Shake or stir to remix.

Note: Did you know that when using dried herbs, it is wise to crush them with your fingers slightly before adding to your other ingredients so that their lovely flavor is released?

A little bit about spices and herbs: Spices and herbs are an excellent way to add big flavor to your meals without adding a lot of fat, calories, or other unwanted ingredients. Remember how the food chemists work on foods? If something is low-fat, look out for it to be high in sugar or high in salt. If it's low-sodium, it may be high in fat or high in sugar. The big three generally can't be removed from a food altogether without losing taste completely.

And, it turns out, herbs and spices can add a healthy boost to your foods too. Why don't you see more of them in packaged or processed foods? Instead, you'll see things like "natural flavors" or "imitation flavorings" on the label. Spices or herbs don't always have the long shelf life that packaged food producers would like. They might also add extra cost to the manufacturing process, which makes them unappealing for the bottom line. However, when you buy fresh herbs, or even dried herbs, you can season your meals for just pennies.

Certain spices, such as cinnamon, have high amounts of antioxidants called *polyphenols*, a plant compound that can lower inflammation in the body and is thought to fight against damage from free radicals. Other herbs and spices that have high evidence of health benefits are thyme, turmeric, chili peppers, garlic, oregano, basil, and rosemary.

ORZO BASIL VEGGIE SIDE

Are you a basil lover? Whether it is green or red, we just love its flavor. Those fresh little leaves can boost your immune system, and may improve production of infection-fighting antibodies up to 20 percent. "The unique array of active constituents called flavonoids found in basil provide protection at the cellular level. Orientin and vicenin are two water-soluble flavonoids that have been of particular interest in basil and in studies on human white blood cells; these components of basil protect cell structures as well as chromosomes from radiation and oxygen-based damage.

"In addition, basil has been shown to provide protection against unwanted bacterial growth. These anti-bacterial properties of basil are not associated with its unique flavonoids, but instead with its volatile oils, which contain estragole, linalool, cineole, eugenol, sabinene, myrcene, and limonene."[32]

---

32 *World's Healthiest Foods*, "Basil Article," WHFoods.com, http://www. whfoods.com/genpage.php?tname=foodspice&dbid=85 (Accessed 19 October 2013)

The addition of herbs is just wonderful to enhance the "mundane" veggies you may have in your fridge. We use broccoli, sun-dried tomatoes, lots of garlic, and mushrooms, but you can use just about any veggie you like. If you are diabetic, you may have noticed that the veggies we use are virtually "free." The only carbohydrates you are adding are the small amount of pasta and olive oil. This healthy side shouldn't throw you for a curve!

INGREDIENTS:
   ½ cup uncooked orzo
   ¼ cup sun-dried tomatoes, diced
   1 teaspoon garlic, minced
   ¼ fresh basil, chopped
   1 tablespoon white balsamic vinegar
   1 cup broccoli, cut into florets
   1 cup mushrooms, sliced
   Nuts or seeds of your choice

INSTRUCTIONS:
In a saucepan prepare the orzo according to the package directions and cook for about eight minutes (it should be just a little underdone as it will be added to your skillet). Heat a skillet over medium heat and swirl in 1 ½ tablespoons olive oil. Add the sun-dried tomato and garlic and stir-fry to infuse the oil with these flavors for about two minutes. Lower the heat and stir-fry the mushrooms just until they lose just a bit of their moisture and are lightly cooked. Drain the orzo and add it to the skillet with the chopped basil, vinegar, and your vegetables. Return to the low heat and roll the orzo and veggies in the flavored oil. We like our veggies bright green and barely cooked so that they retain all their nutrients.

Serve with a lean protein such as all white meat chicken or fish and you will have a fast and easy meal quickly prepared.

CHIA SEEDS HELP WITH CHOLESTEROL

All you have to do is turn on the TV and you'll know that millions of people have a cholesterol problem. Major drug companies can't seem to advertise their pharmaceuticals enough! However, if the idea of spending loads of money on prescriptions every month—while risking side effects—isn't something you enjoy, it might be time to look for another, healthier solution. Many cholesterol problems can be solved through the food choices you make.

You might have also noticed that statin drugs have come under a negative light in some studies. It's known that they deplete body levels of coenzyme Q10 (CoQ10), which is something your heart needs in order to function correctly. They can also deplete other critical nutrients from the body and sometimes lower good cholesterol as well. Sure, you can supplement with CoQ10 pills, but that's even more money out of your pocket! So, aside from all the expense, do you really want to risk these negative effects?

The good news is that you can lower your cholesterol naturally and inexpensively through food. You may have seen the claims on famous products like Cheerios and Quaker Oats that soluble fiber combined with a low saturated fat diet may reduce the risk of heart disease. There's more to it than that, and it's all beneficial to you!

A low-fat diet is great, but you also need some proactive cholesterol cleaners in your corner if you really want to beat down the threat of hardening arteries and cholesterol clogs. The key isn't to avoid all fats or cholesterol sources because your body actually needs some to function properly. It's the ability to sweep away the bad and encourage the good that will lead to better health.

How can chia put the brakes on such a big problem as cholesterol? There are so many ways and you can examine each one in this book Read on to find out exactly how each fascinating facet benefits you.

First, soluble fiber: The exterior of the chia seed is covered in soluble fiber. But this isn't just any soluble fiber like that of an oat or flax seed. The fiber of chia is special in that it can absorb *nine* times the weight of the seed in water and hold it close to the surface. When it does this, it forms a bead of gel with the consistency of a gelatin snack. This gel isn't easily removed from the seed. It takes the digestive system a while to use and remove it, thus hydrating the colon and easing digestion. When food doesn't linger in the colon as long, the body doesn't get as much of a chance to absorb harmful cholesterol particles from food.

Second, insoluble fiber: Insoluble fiber cannot be digested or absorbed by the body. It is sometimes referred to as roughage and acts as a sweeper in the intestines. When food doesn't sit around or become overly dry in the colon, toxic substances don't build up. Unfriendly bacteria don't get the chance to go to work. When insoluble fiber is taking up space in the digestive system, you're more likely to feel full for longer and thus not eat as much at meal-time. Losing excess weight is another key to keeping cholesterol down.

Third, unsaturated fatty acids: These may sound complicated but they're important for cell respiration (oxygen transported into cells) and the lubrication and resilience of cells. There's an especially important fatty acid that your body can't make; it's called linoleic acid. You usually get this from raw plant-source foods, but who gets enough of those these days? With chia seeds you won't have to worry about it. They're rich in this important nutrient.

How are these important for your cholesterol? They combine with cholesterol in the body to form membranes that hold cells together. It puts cholesterol to good use but only if you have enough of it to make the combination!

Fourth, long-chain triglycerides: These large molecules take a stand to scrub cholesterol off artery walls but only when eaten in the right proportions. Chia seeds have these long-chain triglycerides in the right proportions to help reduce cholesterol for you.

Fifth, risk factors: Reducing or eliminating risk factors for high cholesterol is important as well. Some risk factors such as heredity, you can't do anything about, but others such as obesity and diabetes you can help control with chia. (The soluble fiber in chia seeds helps control blood sugar levels by slowing down the transformation of carbohydrates into sugars.)

Sixth, inflammation: Cholesterol can build up on artery walls as a means of protecting the artery from inflammation. If you reduce inflammation and free-radical damage, you can often reduce cholesterol as well. Inflammation is caused by free radicals (which you can fight with antioxidants), a sugar overload (too much sugar is no good for you), an abundance of overly acidic foods (dairy and sweets are acidic), and pollutants in the food or environment. You may not be able to do anything about pollutants but you are in control of your menu.

It's important to understand that not all fats are bad and that taking in healthy oils is an important part of a balanced diet. There are so many delicious chia seed recipes, including breakfast bars, granola, fruit smoothies, and more, that adding this tiny seed to your diet is a snap.

With the chia seed, you get all the nutrition and all the taste. Remember, "you are what you eat," so eating healthy is a big step toward being healthy. Chia isn't some foreign miracle berry or fruit grown in a far-off land and sold at a premium price either— these seeds cost under $1 per day.

If you're looking for an all-natural, pesticide-free, delicious, and *easy* way to lower your cholesterol, consider adding chia seeds to your diet. You'll be amazed at what they can do for you!

MORE ABOUT CHOLESTEROL: A HEART SURGEON'S CHANGE OF HEART—WHAT HE LEARNED CAN SAVE YOUR LIFE!

You can learn more about cholesterol from Dr. Dwight Lundell. Lundell is the past chief of staff and chief of surgery at Banner Heart Hospital, Mesa, Arizona. He has several quotes in this section, thanks to his extensive cholesterol research. When a heart surgeon who has seen the insides of five thousand people's arteries has a change of heart, it's definitely something to take note of— especially if you want to protect your health and the health of the ones you care for. Lundell actually caught onto something that in hindsight is pretty obvious. However, with his medical expertise, he was able to not only shed more light on the topic but also figure out the all-important *why* of the matter.

The problem is that the answer seems to fly in the face of a lot of common medical knowledge and goes against all sorts of rhetoric the public has been hearing for years. The topic is heart disease, cholesterol, and heart attacks. Heart disease is the number one killer of people in the United States today, and it's likely to keep its top spot, so long as no one changes their diet. Pharmaceutical companies would love cutting cholesterol to be the answer to this problem but what if cholesterol buildup on artery walls was only a *side effect* of something else going on in the body?

To study this further, you need to understand inflammation. *Inflammation* is a body's natural reaction to some harmful substance. A bee sting will certainly cause inflammation of the surrounding tissue until the poison and histamines are removed from the area. Inflammation can be good if only continued for short periods of time. The problem occurs when certain parts of the body are frequently or constantly inflamed. Then, instead of being beneficial, the inflammation turns to harm and can even be deadly.

In the case of the cholesterol side effect, it's the arteries of the body that are under attack from frequent inflammation. Cholesterol is used by the body to coat the arteries and protect them from inflammation. The problem is that this restricts blood flow and can cause dangerous pieces of this coating to break off and cause any number of maladies. This is what people today see: cholesterol as the enemy, building up to "attack" people in various ways.

The root, however, lies deeper. What if you could stop cholesterol from building up? Sure, you could take expensive medicines but wouldn't it be better to fight back at the core cause: inflammation?

You are what you eat. This is a fairly simple illustration and perhaps that's why it's often overlooked. With the abundance of unsaturated fats, vegetable oils, low-fat foods, diets, low-carb alternatives, artificial sweeteners, zero-calorie (i.e., nonwater) drinks, pills, prescriptions, and any number of countless other "health foods," how can obesity and heart disease actually be on the *rise*?

No one can answer that question. If all that stuff really were as good for you as it is claimed to be, everyone today should be super fit. Heart disease should be on its way into the history books, not at the head of the charts. The answer isn't, "Oh, people are ignoring their health and never exercising and they just eat low-nutrition food all the time." Can 60 percent of Americans be that far off-base? (Sixty percent of Americans were considered to be overweight in 2009.[33]) It's very hard to believe that this many people could be so enamored of doing the wrong thing so consistently.

What's the real problem? These low-carb, artificially sweetened, omega-6 oil–rich foods are actually the culprit in causing

33   CDC, "Fast Stats Obesity and Overweight," http://www.cdc.gov/nchs/fastats/overwt.htm (Accessed 19 October 2013)

inflammation in the arteries. The main enemies are simple carbohydrates found in processed foods (these turn to sugars very quickly), refined sugar, and omega-6 oils (oils that when out of balance produce cytokines, the inflammatory molecules).

"What does all this have to do with inflammation? Blood sugar is controlled by the body, in a normal state, in a very narrow range. Extra sugar molecules attach to a variety of proteins that in turn injure the blood vessel wall. This repeated injury to the blood vessel wall sets off inflammation. When you spike your blood sugar level several times a day, every day, it is exactly like taking sandpaper to the inside of your delicate blood vessels,"[34] says Dr. Lundell.[35]

While refined sugar and simple starches may be a bit easier to avoid, what about the omega-6 oil? Your body *does* need some of it for healthy function but it must be balanced with the healthy omega-3 oil. The ideal ratio is more omega-3 than -6. However, with saturated fats, animal fats, and other sources of omega-3 being labeled as "fattening" or "less healthy," the balance has been thrown off. Omega-6 fat also gives foods a longer shelf life, which is best for the bottom line—not you!

The truth is, while omega-6 oils may look attractive on the surface (e.g., soy oil, sunflower oil, corn oil) because of slower spoilage and being unsaturated, they're actually behind a lot of the inflammation that's keeping people at risk and overweight!

Lundell says, "Animal fats contain less than 20 percent omega-6 and are much less likely to cause inflammation than the supposedly healthy oils labeled polyunsaturated. Forget the 'science' that has been drummed into your head for decades. The science that saturated fat alone causes heart disease is nonexistent. The science that saturated fat raises blood cholesterol is also very

34; 35 Scott Net, "Heart Surgeon Speaks Out on What Really Causes Heart Disease," http://www.sott.net/article/242516-Heart-surgeon-speaks-out-on-what-really-causes-heart-disease (Accessed 19 October 2013)

weak. Because we now know that cholesterol is not the cause of heart disease, the concern about saturated fat is even more absurd today."

So what's the good news in all of this? It's not too late! Chances are, if you are reading this you *can* reverse the damage to your artery walls. And you can also prevent more inflammation from occurring in the future. When you cut out inflammation, you also stop the body's need to plaster the artery walls with potentially harmful cholesterol. There are also many delicious solutions and great reasons to raise omega-3 levels.

Omega-3 may actually play a part in weight loss success! Jade Beutler, an author of *Understanding Fats & Oils*, says, "Omega-3 fatty acids are gaining popularity with those looking to lose weight while attaining optimal health, and the latest research has revealed numerous slimming secrets attributed to omega-3s." *USA Weekend* magazine also reported a study wherein overweight dieters who included omega-3s in their eating plans lost two more pounds monthly than the control group who did not include these foods.[36] So, what can you do?

First, eat greener. Try to add more unprocessed foods to your diet. Fresh fruits and vegetables may have carbohydrates, but they are mostly complex carbohydrates. Even in the sweetest fruits, these are broken down more slowly and blood sugar isn't so heavily affected. Stay away from or minimize starchy foods such as white potatoes and white breads. The healthiest food is the food that's closest to its natural state. Grass-fed beef, free-range chicken and turkey, colorful fruits, squash, vegetables, nuts, and seeds are key to stopping inflammation so that your natural healing process can take over.

---

36 *USA Weekend*, "Eat Fats to Lose Weight? Yes. If They're the Right Kind," http://www.usaweekend.com/article/20090208/HEALTH03/91111017/ Eat-fats-lose-weight- (Accessed 19 October 2013)

Want to help balance your omega-3 and omega-6? As you may know, fish and fish oil are rich in healthy omega-3 oils. But what if you don't want fish every night? Don't like the idea of cod-liver oil? Worried about fish absorbing harmful pollutants and spreading them to your family? Or, maybe you want to follow the vegetarian path so that the oceans can recover from overfishing. No matter what your reason is, omega-3 just got a lot healthier and easier to add to your diet with chia seeds.

This tiny seed is nature's richest plant-based source of omega-3 oil. By weight, it is even richer than salmon, so every spoonful of chia can help you tip the balance to the healthy omega-3 side. The best part is that there's no flavor. You can add these seeds to whatever you like (unlike fish!) to get your daily amount of omega-3. They're also full of B vitamins, more calcium than milk, and more magnesium than broccoli, all with the taste of whatever you'd like!

"Food of convenience" is part of the reason for this obesity and cholesterol epidemic. Easier, faster, tastier, and longer-lasting has been the motto. Chia seeds may be the ultimate convenient food. What is easier than sprinkling a spoonful onto something you were going to eat or drink anyway? What is more delicious than the best taste that *you* specify? And what natural, uncooked, preservative-free, and pesticide-free food lasts two years without refrigeration? Nothing else but the chia seed can answer yes to all these questions.

BIG PHARMA VERSUS CHOLESTEROL

Did you know that almost half of Americans take a prescription drug? Melinda Wenner Moyer, writing for *Scientific American* on March 31, 2010, found that "an estimated twenty million Americans take statins, making these cholesterol-lowering drugs the most widely prescribed class in the world. In coming years, these numbers are only expected to increase. In June 2011 the full patent for Pfizer's block-buster Lipitor (atorvastatin) will expire, making the drug significantly more affordable. And later this year in 2010 the National Cholesterol Education Program (NCEP) of the National Heart, Lung, and Blood Institute will release guidelines that could recommend statins for younger people who have no cholesterol issues—a move that they think could stave off cardiovascular disease later in life but also introduces questions about aggressively treating the healthy."[37]

What about the side effects of these medications? What about the long-term health consequences of depleted CoQ10 levels? What about the added expense and stress caused by these supposed recommendations?

Dr. Joseph Mercola, the physician and author, writes, "There's really no reason to take satins and suffer the damaging health effects from these dangerous drugs. The fact is that 75 percent of your cholesterol is produced by your liver, which is influenced by your insulin levels. Therefore, if you optimize your insulin levels, you will automatically optimize your cholesterol. It follows, then, that my primary recommendations for safely regulating your cholesterol have to do with modifying your diet and lifestyle."[38]

It would be more beneficial (but not nearly as profitable for drug manufacturers) to educate both parents and kids on eating a healthy diet. We watched a TED talk where many school-aged children could not identify garden vegetables when displayed in a classroom. They had never seen their parents prepare many of the fruits and veggies. They had no idea how to cook them. Parents are not cooking *and* not cooking with their children to teach

---

37   *Scientific American*, "Static Over Statins: Should Young People Without Cholesterol Problems Take Statins?" http://www.scientificamerican.com/article.cfm?id=static-over-statins (Accessed 19 October 2013)

38   Dr. Joseph Mercola, "Statin Nation: The Great Cholesterol Cover-Up," http://articles.mercola.com/sites/articles/archive/2013/05/11/statin-nation.aspx (Accessed 22 October 2013)

them healthy life skills. Life skills even minimally taught in home economic classes at schools are a thing of the past.

There are some surprising foods that help out with cholesterol. You already know about the benefits of adding fiber, but did you know that cranberries can help out too? How about refreshing citrus zest? According to Prepared Foods Network writer Angela Stokes, citrus peels may contribute to lower risks of heart disease. A study published in the *Journal of Agriculture and Food Chemistry* found that the PMF compounds (polymethoxylated flavones) in citrus peels have the potential to lower cholesterol when included in your diet.[39] You'll notice citrus zest in various recipes throughout this book. When you use zest, you improve the flavor—and the healthiness—of the dish!

CRANBERRY WATERMELON SMOOTHIE

Do you know how splendid cranberries are for your body? Cranberries are loaded with vitamin C and antioxidants and have an antibacterial effect on the body. Cranberry juice is often used to fight the bacteria that can cause urinary tract infections. Cranberries are also good for cardiovascular health. They help with the prevention of the oxidation of LDL cholesterol, which may help prevent atherosclerosis. A study was also done wherein cranberries improved blood vessel function in people who already had atherosclerosis.[40]

The problem with winter holiday cranberry sauces is the amount of sugar added to them. So, make the sweetness a natural sugar, like in this smoothie with watermelon and banana.

---

39   Angela Stokes, "Citrus Peel Benefits," LiveStrong.com, http://www.livestrong.com/article/155590-citrus-peel-benefits/ (Accessed 19 October 2013)

40   Reed J., "Cranberry Flavonoids, Atherosclerosis and Cardiovascular Health," Pub Med, http://www.ncbi.nlm.nih.gov/pubmed/12058989 (Accessed 19 October 2013)

INGREDIENTS:

    ½ cup fresh or frozen cranberries
    1 cup watermelon chunks
    ½ banana
    1 teaspoon chia

INSTRUCTIONS:

In your mini-chopper or blender, add the fresh or defrosted cranberries and chop until finely cut. Add the banana, chia, and watermelon. Blend. Don't forget that a blender is not a calorie eliminator. Many people will have "a smoothie and . . ." because the smoothie is "just a drink." Whatever you blend in with your smoothie, you're still getting all of the calories of the original fruits or vegetables. That's why chia is an important addition here: it makes the drink fill you up so you can easily have "just a drink" and still feel satisfied until your next meal.

BANANA ALMOND BREAKFAST BITES

Eating breakfast in the morning is always a good idea. If you skip breakfast or just have a cup of coffee, you're more likely to gain weight, which never helps with cholesterol. People who pick up a healthy breakfast with a little protein, a little fiber, and a little fruit have been shown to have an easier time losing weight.

These breakfast bites are a great idea for busy mornings. You can grab a bite on your way out the door and the protein from the almond butter and chia seeds will help keep you energized until lunch. These are also gluten-free! Oats provide fiber and the banana provides sweetness, so that you don't feel deprived or bland in the morning. There's more fiber here than in white-flour toaster pastries, fried doughnuts, or sugar-loaded muffins that might as well be cupcakes. The fruity, nutty taste is even something kids can enjoy!

Ideally, for breakfast you should have a veggie and fruit smoothie, a beautifully prepared omelet, or a cup of Greek yogurt with berries. That's the family life on TV. In real life, the dog threw up on the carpet, the baby has diarrhea, and you don't know where your car keys are! When time is shorter than usual and you need to have a little something to break your fast, try making a batch of these oat and almond bites on the weekend. These bites are easy and fast and can be used as a grab-and-go snack for everyone at any time; just don't grab too many!

INGREDIENTS:

¾ cup flour

¾ cup quick-cooking oats

½ cup almond nut butter (with no sugar added, and stirred to combine the oil)

¼ cup sugar

¼ teaspoon baking soda

Dash salt

½ teaspoon cinnamon

2 tablespoons chia gel

½ cup smashed banana

1 egg

Sliced almond chips for garnish, if desired (about 1 or 2 per cookie)

INSTRUCTIONS:

Preheat the oven to 400 degrees Fahrenheit. Then, in a measuring cup, smash a portion of a banana to equal half a cup. Next, in a medium bowl, combine the flour, oats, sugar, soda, salt, and cinnamon. Place the smashed banana, the almond butter, the egg, and the chia gel into the bowl and stir to combine. Drop a heavily rounded teaspoonful onto a cookie sheet coated with cooking spray. Bake for twelve to fifteen minutes until the bottoms are lightly browned. Once the cookies have cooled, store them in an airtight container. These cookies also freeze well.

A REAL EDIBLE SOLUTION FOR PICKY-EATING KIDS

Any parent who has a picky kid has not only a hassle (what to cook, and what to serve?) but also legitimate nutrition concerns. With the amount of refined foods that are packed with additives and artificial flavors, colors, and so forth, as well as unhealthy choices overwhelming the marketplace and school lunchroom, it can look like an impossible task to get the right nutrients into your child's diet.

If your dinner table is the scene of a huge fight or you make a trip to the fast-food restaurant more often than not, you might need a little help from the chia seed! Finally, there's a safe, easy way to get kids to have the nutrition they need. And, best of all, it tastes like whatever your kids want it to!

As you know, the flavor of food is often the biggest hurdle for picky eaters. "It tastes gross!" "This smells terrible!" "I'm not eating *that*." This can make variety impossible or deprive kids of a vegetable with powerful nutrients just because it tastes terrible. (Broccoli, anyone?) But what if you could ensure that your kids got

- Magnesium: fifteen times more than broccoli
- Calcium: six times more than whole milk
- Omega-3: nearly nine times the amount found in salmon
- Fiber: more than flax seed and two times more than bran flakes
- Iron: nearly three times more than spinach
- Protein: more than soy (chia has 2 grams of protein for every 10 grams of seeds, while tofu products generally have 1 gram per every 10 grams of product)
- Cholesterol: none (unlike fish)

So, what is this super solution that can give everything from a yummy milkshake to a bowl of cereal as much nutritional kick as vegetables?

Chia seeds.

For example, if you add a spoonful of chia to yogurt and stir, the seeds will take on the taste of the yogurt as the seeds hydrate. They do not add their own flavor or take away the flavor of the yogurt so you don't have to worry about the yogurt tasting different once you add the seeds. The same goes for baked goods. You can pour them into pancakes, muffins, breads, or anything your kids love. The flavorless seeds go down easy because they taste just like what they're in.

When you have chia in the house, your days of worrying whether your kids are getting enough protein when all they want to eat is mac'n cheese are over! The protein is complete too (like that found in meat). So, until your kids' tastes grow up, you don't have to worry as much about their nutrition. Don't let them fill up on junk food or fast food; take control of your family's nutrition now for a healthy lifetime later. There are plenty of kid-friendly recipes you can find right here in this book and online with search engines to get your family started easily.

APPLE AND MELON CHIA SALAD

Are you having trouble getting your kids to eat salad? Do they only want ranch dressing on their pile of leaves, if they will eat it at all? This lively salad may just be your salvation! Fruits and veggies and just a little light dressing may tickle their taste buds. They may decide to "get off the ranch" and vacation in Variety City.

INGREDIENTS:

FOR THE SALAD:

About 2 handfuls of dark greens of your choice

1 large green apple, chopped (with the peel left on)

About ¼ of an average size cantaloupe, cut into bite-size pieces

1 average size cucumber (deseeded and peeled), cut into bite-size pieces

2 tablespoons chopped red onion

¼ cup dried cranberries

¼ cup nuts of your choice

FOR THE DRESSING:

1 tablespoon agave nectar or honey

1 lemon, zested and juiced

1 tablespoon olive oil

1 teaspoon chia seeds

½ teaspoon Dijon mustard

INSTRUCTIONS:

In a large bowl place the prepared veggies and fruits. In a small container mix the dressing and pour it over all the fruits and veggies. Watch in amazement when this salad gets gobbled up! You can tailor your salad to your family's tastes. Are pears in season? Would little chunks of Swiss cheese or cheddar cheese be a treat?

CHIA BROCCOLI-ORANGE SIDE

Don't like broccoli? This side salad might change your mind. How we taste things depends mostly on the quantity and type of taste receptors we are born with. These receptors are clustered within the taste buds on the tongue and react to sweet, salty, sour, and bitter foods. Broccoli sometimes sets off the bitter receptors too much making some people hate the taste, but you can trick taste buds by adding a little something sweet at the same time!

Here, the orange sections lend a little bit of fruit sugars to the salad, which can trick taste buds into accepting broccoli. Why should you want to accept broccoli? Raw broccoli is loaded with vitamin C, fiber, protein, potassium, and vitamin A. "Cooking broccoli too long destroys the enzyme myrosinase, which helps convert broccoli's cancer-fighting compound sulforaphane into its active form," reports *LiveStrong.com*[41]

This recipe is only slightly warmed, so you keep the nutrients where they belong: in the broccoli!

Ingredients:

2 cups broccoli florets

½ of a 15.5 ounce can cannellini beans, rinsed and drained

1 small sweet red pepper, diced

1 naval orange

1 tablespoon chia gel

1 pinch paprika

INSTRUCTIONS:

Place the florets in a microwaveable bowl with a tablespoon of water and cover. Cook for forty-five to sixty seconds. Zest and section a naval orange, retaining the juice in a small cup. Add the cannellini beans, red pepper, zest, and orange sections. Pour the orange juice and chia gel over the veggies. Sprinkle a dash of paprika over the veggies, cover, and microwave for twenty to thirty seconds.

Let's change some minds about broccoli!

COOL GREEN CHIA GAZPACHO

When it is a about a "bazillion" degrees outside and no one feels like cooking, this cold and fresh-tasting soup may just keep you from wilting away! It is so easy and just requires a blender. A gazpacho soup is traditionally served cold and is comprised of chunky, raw

---

41   Becky Miller, "Raw Vegetables vs. Cooked Vegetables," LiveStrong.com, http://www.livestrong.com/article/58058-raw-vegetables-vs.-cooked-vegetables/#ixzz2iMrenk4Z (Accessed 19 October 2013)

vegetables which include tomato, onion, and spicy peppers. The following recipe is a cool, almost sweet, green gazpacho that may keep you and your family from melting. Serve with your favorite sandwich, and no cooking for you!

INGREDIENTS:

2 large handfuls of fresh spinach (with larger stems removed)

1 ½ cups white grape juice (Read the ingredient label! No high fructose corn syrup please.)

1 cup vegetable broth

1 small cucumber, peeled and deseeded

1 small zucchini, peeled and cut up

1 rib of celery, cut into large pieces

1 lime, zested and ready for juicing

1 tablespoon dry chia

1 cup green, seedless grapes, cut in half

Pour about one half-cup of the white grape juice into the blender and add the spinach leaves. Puree until the spinach is finely chopped. Pour the contents into a medium bowl. Next, add the cucumber, zucchini, and celery, adding grape juice as needed. These veggies just need a pulse or two as you want them to be in small pieces. You may have to work in batches depending on the size of your blender or chopper. As you blend, add the veggies to the medium bowl with the spinach.

Stir in the chia, juice the lime, and add the lime zest and the grapes along with the vegetable broth. Cover and chill in the fridge for several hours. This is a "starter" soup, or a small cup of accompanying soup—not a *big* bowl of soup.

We garnish this soup with radish slices. Do a taste test; if you like your soup a little zippy, add a few radishes to the blender and stir them into the soup. Got a picky eater? The sweetness of the grape juice disguises the spinach and this gazpacho will be a total hit. You'll hear, "Let's have this again, really, really soon!"

Chia Seeds and Hydration

Do you know how much of your body is water? About three-quarters of your weight is water! By the time you feel thirsty, you most likely are on the road to being dehydrated. Some drinks (e.g., alcohol and caffeine) can actually work to help keep you dehydrated. By drinking the right type of drinks, you can not only stay hydrated but also improve your health. When every sip is a chance to add nutrients and improve digestion, you can get excited about staying hydrated. Almost all systems require water to run efficiently, just look at this list:

- Blood (mostly water)
- Gastric juices (mostly water-based)
- Your eyes and tears (mostly water)
- Saliva (mostly water)
- Spinal fluid (mostly water)
- Synovial fluid around the joints (mostly water)
- Skin's elasticity (dependent on water)
- Bodily waste removal (dependent on, and mostly, water)

If you are not drinking enough water, you are creating a hostile environment that causes all your body's systems to work inefficiently and unhappily. Feel tired? Drink water. Just a little thirsty? Drink water. Five liters of your blood is counting on water. Your blood needs to deliver nutrients and oxygen to all of your tissues, all day, every day. Make eliminating the toxins and waste products from your body a top priority. When your digestive system is in top shape, you can more easily deal with environmental pollutants, bad bacteria, and the harmful byproducts of digestion.

Did you know that liquid calories in soft drinks are the biggest source of added sugar in today's diets? Soft drinks can be quite addictive, and the caffeine in sodas just compounds the addictive properties. Add about two hundred-plus calories on top of your normal daily calorie intake, and, "whoops," that is 73,000 additional sugar-laden calories, or about twenty pounds of extra weight, per year.

You might say, "Ah, but I drink diet soda! I'm tricking my body."

Nope! Artificial sweeteners disrupt the normal hormonal and neurological signals that control hunger and the "I'm full" feeling. Many scientific studies have shown that they lead to weight gain rather than weight loss. Some people's reaction to aspartame actually includes inducing hunger every time they consume it.

So, what is the alternative to sweetened sodas, high-fructose "fruit juices" made from 10 percent real fruit, or faux vitamin waters? Water—clean, filtered, pure water. Our bodies are composed of about 96 percent water. Make your own "vitamin" water with a wedge of lime or lemon and chia. Mull a few strawberries and add water or seltzer and chia gel. Once you get away from soda for a week or two, you may notice that the next time you try it, it tastes way too sweet. It was always that sweet! You just didn't notice because you were desensitized to the sweetness.

What about high fructose corn syrup (HFCS)?

It permeates just about everything! Take a look at the ingredient list of products that you wouldn't even think should be sweet at all. For instance, it's in salad dressings, savory sauces, and so much more. You'll find that it's especially common in fruit juice bottles, cans of juice concentrate, sports drinks, and health waters, and even added to some "fresh-squeezed" juices too. HFCS and cane or beet sugar are not biochemically identical or processed the same way by the body.

The Corn Refiners Association has produced commercials stating that it is OK in moderation, and that's true. However, most people can't get it in moderation because it's in so many processed foods and almost all of the flavored beverages you can find on store shelves.

However, don't think that you just have to drink plain, boring water! There are many nonwater drinks for you to choose from to keep your menu entertaining. Staying hydrated does not have to be a chore. There are so many healthy drinks you can choose from, including water with a squeeze of fresh lemon or lime; green, black, or chai tea; water with a shot of fresh fruit juice added; mulled fresh fruit; or minted water.

You can use ready-made flavoring liquids or flavoring powders, as long as they don't contain artificial sweeteners such as aspartame or sucralose. You will see more options with natural sweeteners such as stevia (derived from a leaf) or xylitol (derived from tree bark). Caffeine and sugar or sugar substitutes are the biggest culprits for stressing your pancreas and liver. Also, aspartame can have the side effect of making some people hungrier! Drinking "diet" sodas or diet fruit drinks can actually sabotage a diet much faster than can any sugar-loaded drink.

Sweetener choices: When you make chia drinks at home, you don't have to worry about the choice of sweeteners. Agave nectar is low on the glycemic index (certainly lower than cane or beet sugar or high fructose corn syrup). It has more calories than regular sugars, but it is 40 percent sweeter, so you end up using less to get the same result.

Agave also has saponins that kill bad bacteria while promoting the good bacteria that help you digest foods. Agave also has inulin fiber. This special type of fiber sooths the digestive tract and has been reported to help ease the symptoms of irritable bowel and colitis.

Stevia is two hundred times sweeter than sugar, but has a glycemic index of zero. It's also a zero-calorie food. A Japanese study recently found that stevia can strengthen bones and increase their mineral density.[42] Certain kinds of bad bacteria also hate stevia as well, so this sweet leaf is definitely something you should consider.

When you choose a healthy drink, you cut your beloved organs a break! If you're stuck on soda, experiment with as many different drink flavors as you possibly can. Try each type of tea (iced and hot), and don't be afraid to add fruit juice to plain water (a little fruit juice is fine; a glass of it contains more calories and more sugar than you need). Sparkling water with lemon, lime, orange, or your favorite fruit added can also be a great substitute for soda, as the "fizz factor" is still there.

What about alkaline water? You might have heard about alkaline water. It can either be processed to be more alkaline than normal, pH-neutral water, or it can come from a natural spring that was alkaline to begin with. Some people find the taste of alkaline water to be extremely refreshing. If you have never tried alkaline water, give it a shot! It could totally change your opinion on "plain, boring water." Try for a pH of about 8 to 8.8. If the water is too alkaline, it may slow down your digestion if you drink it with a meal.

What does chia do to help keep you hydrated? Soluble fiber is the key to staying hydrated with chia seeds. Soluble fiber can prolong hydration and retain electrolytes in body fluids, especially during exertion or exercise. (So try the chia sports drink recipe in this book!) When you have normal fluid retention during exercise, or during times when it's really hot out (i.e., you're sweating from just walking around in the sun or the heat), soluble fiber ensures

---

42   Jami Cooley, RN CNWC, "Stevia Benefits Bone Health And More," Article Part Two, *Natural Health Advisory Daily*, http://www.naturalhealthadvisory.com/daily/osteoporosis-prevention-and-treatment/natural-sugar-substitute-stevia-benefits-bone-health-and-more/ (Accessed 19 October 2013)

electrolyte dispersion across cell membranes. When you maintain your hydration levels, fluid balances in your body can keep up with normal cellular function during exertion. Gelled chia seeds can be easily digested and absorbed. When something's easy to digest, you get the nutrients into your cells faster, ready for use on your next big play, a trip to the gym, or just a jog outdoors.

As we have been hearing for years, by drinking and staying hydrated you will make your brain (mostly water) and bodily systems (mostly water) work more smoothly. Your goal: the best *you*!

It's time to get started with better hydration! You can use these recipes for great chia drinks to help keep you hydrated longer and happy. You don't need to feel flavor deprived.

CHIA FRESCA

The drink that started it all!

Chia fresca has been enjoyed in Mexico for hundreds of years. Because the chia plant loves the hot, dry climate there, chia has always been readily available. The people learned that you can fill up, add electrolytes (great for hot weather workouts), and hydrate the digestive system by drinking chia gel. Chia fresca is traditionally made with chia seeds, filtered water, lime juice, and a sweetening agent, such as agave nectar, sugar cane juice, or honey. A quick stirring helps the chia blend the flavors, then the cool, refreshing beverage is ready to enjoy. This recipe makes two eight-ounce glasses.

INGREDIENTS:
    16 ounces filtered water
    6 tablespoon lime juice (fresh-squeezed, about 2 limes)
    1 tablespoon chia seeds
    Your choice of sweetener

INSTRUCTIONS:

To keep this healthy, use a sugar alternative such as stevia, xylitol, monk fruit, or even agave nectar. Agave is sweeter than sugar, so you can use less of it. Stevia, xylitol, and monk fruit (lo han guo) are all zero-calorie sweeteners that taste sweet, but the body does not recognize them as a sugar. The key to this drink is sweetening it to your taste preference.

CHIA HOT TEA

Chia gel works in hot or cold beverages. If you enjoy hot tea, but want something that will also fill you up, consider adding chia gel. Many teas are excellent for your health. Did you know that green tea has compounds that help guard your DNA against age-related damage? Chia has free-radical fighters too, such as the dark-colored anthocyanins in the seed shells.

If you have a tea infuser, add orange zest to the loose-leaf green tea. Don't have an infuser? Add a tablespoon of orange juice for a fresh citrus zing. To make this tea, use green tea, orange juice (or zest), one-quarter teaspoon cinnamon, and one-quarter teaspoon ground cloves. This makes about two eight-ounce cups of tea.

COLD FRUIT CHIA TEAS

Chia hot tea is good, and chia cold tea is just as great! Unsweetened tea bags are easy to use in flavors such as raspberry, blueberry, lemon, and citrus. There are more great fruit-flavored teas on the shelves right now than ever before. Add chia gel and you have a fantastic cold drink that also fills you up. Brew the tea, let it cool, then chill and add chia gel. Sweeten these teas with a sprinkle of stevia and they'll appeal to kids too because of their fruity flavors. It's so easy because you can make a whole pitcher of tea ahead of time and then add as much gel as you want to the glass when you're ready to drink. It's so much healthier than soda or diet soda.

CHIA MINI FRUIT DRINKS

You can make your own delicious, inexpensive (compared to store brands!) chia fruit drinks when you use filtered water and frozen fruit juice mix. Be sure to select brands with "pure fruit" because several varieties can have artificial sweeteners or high fructose corn syrup added. Sweetened fruit drinks can have as much sugar as the same amount of soda, so it's important to watch labels so that you know just what you're getting. These drinks are thick like the bottled chia drinks you find in stores, only they cost a whole lot less because you make them at home! Save money and customize the flavors just how you like with these recipes.

Looking for a sweet snack in the afternoon?

Instead of reaching for chips or a candy bar, why not mix up a little four-ounce chia drink?

INGREDIENTS:

    1 tablespoon blueberry pomegranate concentrate
    2 tablespoons filtered water
    3 tablespoons gelled chia seeds
    1 tablespoon lemonade concentrate
    3 tablespoons water
    3 tablespoons gelled chia seeds
    1 teaspoon lime juice (unsweetened)

INSTRUCTIONS:

This will satisfy your sweet tooth while keeping you feeling full until dinnertime. The complete protein in chia will also help with any afternoon energy slumps. Not only is it healthy; it's a big money saver too when you're not spending on energy drinks, fancy coffees, candy, or vending snacks.

MAKE YOUR OWN SPORTS DRINK

Do you know just how much sugar is in typical, store-bought sports drinks? They're loaded! Most twenty-ounce drinks can have about seven or more teaspoons of sugar. You're drinking these rehydrators to replenish the water and nutrients that you lost through sweating for exercise. Lots of sugar doesn't help your exercise efforts. You can avoid these ovesweetened beverages by making your own sports drinks easily at home! Pack them for the big game or the big meet in BPA-free, reusable bottles for even more health benefits.

Most commercially produced sports drinks do exactly what they claim: they help rehydrate your body. The electrolytes (salt, potassium, and magnesium) are lost through sweating, your body's cooling system. Why not make your own sports drink? You can tailor it to your liking with the amount of sweet, tart flavor from your favorite citrus fruit. This make-at-home drink will be far less expensive, fresh, and ready to rehydrate you just as well, without all the sugar, artificial flavors, dyes, or artificial sweeteners.

INGREDIENTS:
    1 quart filtered water
    ¼ cup fresh citrus juice (lemon, lime, or orange)
    ¼ teaspoon salt
    2 or 3 teaspoons agave nectar or honey
    1 tablespoon chia gel

INSTRUCTIONS:
Simply stir to mix everything together. You can add citrus zest for extra tang or to combine flavors. (Make lemon-lime drink, etc.)

Citrus zest is an excellent antioxidant loaded with vitamin C. If you're going to juice the fruits, you might as well zest them too.

When you stay hydrated during outdoor activities, you'll feel better, you'll perform better, and your body will get more benefits from the exercise. Citrus juice is considered an acid but it converts to an alkaline once you drink it.

Note: Did you know? Dave Patania of Eyewitness News of Indianapolis writes,

"A twenty-ounce Powerade weighs in with over seven teaspoons of sugar. Powerade's low-sugar option—just over one. A thirty-two-ounce Gatorade—a staggering fourteen teaspoons of sugar. Gatorade's lower-sugar brand, Propel sixteen ounces, only one and a half teaspoons. A twenty-ounce Vitamin Water tips the scales with just over seven teaspoons."[43]

WATERMELON REFRESHER CHIA SLUSHY

Looking for a great healthy way to cool down in the summer months? Watermelon may be mostly water, but it still manages to pack in a surprising amount of nutrients. Watermelon has potassium (which can be lost during outdoor activities, so it's a good idea to replenish your potassium as you rehydrate), vitamin A, vitamin C, and magnesium too. Watermelons (like tomatoes) contain lots of healthy lycopene, which is good for your cardiovascular and bone health.

INGREDIENTS:

2 cups watermelon chunks
1 tablespoon dry chia
½ cup crushed ice

---

43 Dave Patania, "How Much Sugar Does Your Sports Drink Really Have?," WTHR Indiana's News Leader Eyewitness News, http://www.wthr.com/global/Story.asp?s=7049458 (Accessed 20 October 2013)

Squirt of lime juice

Sparkling water or seltzer

INSTRUCTIONS:

In your blender, pulse to chop the watermelon chunks. Be careful not to reduce it to liquid. Add the chia to hydrate and wait about ten minutes. Add a squirt of lime juice, the crushed ice, and your amount of sparkling water. Pulse once to combine. Now you're ready to pour a glass of sweet, cool, refreshment.

CHIA SEEDS FOR EXERCISE

People who don't "move it" don't lose it. Studies show that exercise can alter your DNA by having a positive effect on your telomeres, which are the protective caps on your chromosomes. With a little exercise you will be healthier and look younger. Exercise will speed up your metabolism and calorie-burning ability. You can enhance your endurance and build strength. You are never too old to build your strength and increase your bone density.

You may think that you are on the go all day long, but you may be surprised. You sat while driving, you sat at your desk, you "watched" the kids, you were not really engaged in very active muscle moving and strengthening. Don't have the time or money to join a gym? No worries! Just do a fast walk around the block, dance in your living room, ride your bike, or run up and down the stairs a couple of times. If you can't find time for cardio (a sustained, elevated heart-rate workout for about twenty minutes or more is "cardio"), good news! Recent studies are showing that a quick blast of exercise (e.g., a sprint twice a day) has really positive effects on physical fitness! You don't have to spend a ton of time exercising to get a benefit.

Borrow a library book with strength-building, low-stress yoga exercises. Yoga can be extremely simple to do. There are sitting yoga exercises, and very simple poses that almost anyone can do. Don't be fooled or intimidated by the super flexible people you see on TV. Yoga is excellent for balance and flexibility. Because there is such a wide range of poses, you can start really simple and build up your flexibility and balance as well as strength at a pace that's right for you.

You will feel happier, feel less stressed, and sleep better when you add a little exercise to your day. If you work up a sweat, that's OK too. Sweating removes waste products from the body. If you're stressed, exercising can use up some of the stress hormones and help calm you down. Even something like walking can help out with intestine function as well. Exercising encourages the digestive system to move food through it a little bit faster.

Chia can help you stay hydrated during exercise. Chia seeds have more potassium by weight than a banana. Potassium helps you keep your electrolyte balance in check while exercising. Chia also hydrates the digestive system. Why not try the make-at-home chia sports drink in this book?

The modern Tarahumara natives of Mexico are known to use chia on their amazing marathon runs. They run through their high-altitude desert homeland while supplementing with chia seeds and water. A quick Internet search for "Tarahumara" will show you the facts about their amazing feats. The ancient Aztecs also used chia on their various army marches through harsh terrain. The seeds were light and easy to carry but very nutritious.

When you exercise, you are doing something great for yourself. If you lift and carry your groceries, your kids, your laundry, and so on, that's a great start at weight-bearing exercises. As time permits, maybe you can add more activities to your list of *fun* things to do. Choosing a physical activity that appeals to you is the most important thing to do. If something's boring or feels like a chore, you're not likely to keep up with it. Some people love running outdoors, while it bores others to tears (or the weather is always bad, or it's too polluted, etc.). There are so many exercise options for all different levels of physical fitness that there's every reason to experiment around to find something you like to do.

It's important to not get too uptight about an eating or exercise routine. Making something healthy into a chore is a good way to get "turned off" from it. If you wanted to run, but it rains, try a bit of yoga stretching instead. If you skip a day, don't freak out. Getting upset over an interruption never helps. It's finding balance in healthy food (with a few treats!) and moving your body in healthy ways that will keep you happier and healthier.

CHIA AND SLEEP: THE ZZZZZ POWER

We are not machines and do not run on batteries that keep going and going. "During sleep we regenerate, which includes growth of new heart and brain cells," states Dr. Matthew Edlund,[44] the director of the Center for Circadian Medicine in Florida. If you are not getting enough sleep for your body's needs, your body can't rejuvenate, and you may feel lethargic. "If people don't sleep enough, they tend to gain weight," Edlund says. Why? Partial sleep deprivation (sleeping fewer than seven hours a night) causes glucose levels to increase. On a regular basis, this leads to insulin resistance, which can cause fat deposits in the abdomen. Sleep also helps control hunger hormones. Consistently getting enough sleep, combined with exercise and a healthy diet, can help you control your weight.[45]

---

44   Dr. Matthew Edlund, "The Rejuvenating Power of Rest," *Huffington Post*, http://www.huffingtonpost.com/matthew-edlund-md/the-rejuvenating-power-of_b_430021.html (Accessed 20 October 2013)

45   Dr Matthew Edlund, "Get Proper Sleep To Keep Your Weight on Point," *USA Weekend*, http://www.usaweekend.com/print/article/20100824/PARTNERS05/308240003/Get-proper-sleep-to-keep-your-weight-on-point (Accessed 22 October 2013)

Canadian researchers looked at the relationship between sleep and weight gain over six years and found that people who slept five to six hours a night gained about four and one-half pounds more than those who rested for seven to eight hours. Light sleepers were also 27 percent more likely to develop obesity than regular sleepers.[46] Sleep is important.

Many people go to bed hungry or with the "munchies" and then have trouble sleeping. There is a way to fix that! Make yourself a chia fresca about twenty minutes before retiring. Turn off all your electronic devices, sip your fresca, relax, and let your natural melatonin work its magic. Chia also has a little tryptophan, an amino acid that helps make serotonin. Serotonin is important for brain health and healthy sleeping habits. The chia will fill your tummy and the alkalizing lime or lemon will set the stage for the repair work that is about to begin while you are sleeping. Rest helps regulate your hunger hormones, ghrelin and leptin. Lack of sleep can stimulate your appetite and may not quiet those pesky voices that say, "Hey! It's snack time."

Omega-3 is also good for sleep, and chia has this great oil! A lack of omega-3 oils can disturb your sleep. When you don't have enough omega-3, your circadian clock is weakened and you're more likely to be a light sleeper (i.e., almost anything can disrupt your rest). Omega-3 oil enhances the secretion of melatonin too, which is important because it helps regulate the wake-sleep cycle. You might have heard of melatonin being used to combat insomnia and jet lag. Make sure that your omega-3 levels are high enough to promote the synthesis and release of these healthy, sleep-helping chemicals in the body.

Note that not everyone can or "should" have eight hours of sleep. Some people don't require it but other people do.

---

46   *My Health News Daily*, "Sleep Is Important to Weight Loss, Research Suggests," http://www.livescience.com/36652-sleep-weight-loss-advice.html (Accessed 20 October 2013)

New baby? Sick child? Crisis in the family or work? Life happens. It may seem that this situation may never end and you'll need to hibernate for a year, but it will. Do the best you can with erratic sleep patterns and know you'll get back to the "sweet spot" on your sleep hours. If you stress out over lack of your ideal hours, it just adds more havoc to your body. Remember college — did you get a "straight eights"?

ALKALINE VERSUS ACIDIC DIETS

Did you know that your body's general ideal pH level is about 7.02? Your blood pH should be slightly alkaline (7.35–7.45). If you go too far above or too far below the range, you open yourself up to diseases and symptoms. A pH of 7.0 is neutral. A pH below 7.0 is acidic. A pH above 7.0 is alkaline.

What are the symptoms of being too acidic? Symptoms can range from dry hair and nails, muscle aches, mouth sores, picking up every cold that comes your way, yeast infections, low energy, cardiovascular conditions, bladder problems, kidney stones, and more. It's a lengthy list, and there's more than just these listed symptoms. If you suspect you might be too acidic, or if you have an annoying symptom that just won't go away, it's a good idea to check your pH. If your liver and pancreas are overburdened by too much acid and not enough alkaline, these organs can't effectively neutralize or eliminate the acid and it builds up in your cells.

How does your body try to neutralize acid? If an alkaline food product is not being digested or there are no reserves of alkaline minerals present in the digestive system, your body will remove alkaline substances from their storage spaces. Your long-term alkaline stores are in your bones and muscles. Calcium and magnesium are the most minerals stolen, which can start you on the way to bone loss and cramping muscles. That's why it's time to think twice about cow's milk. Sure, it has calcium, but it reacts in the body as an acidifier. Does your milk have enough calcium to neutralize itself?

By adding more alkaline foods to your menu, and combining acidifying and alkalinizing foods together (e.g., a pasta salad with a spinach base and spicy orzo and a veggie mix top), you can help keep your body in balance. There are some surprising sources of acid as well as alkaline that are probably already on your menu. For instance, orzo (and all pasta) is acidic. So are healthy items like beans, quinoa, blueberries, cranberries, and avocado oil. These *are* healthy foods, don't give them up! Just have some alkaline foods around to balance them out.

Wait, why isn't a lemon or a lime on this acid food list? What about meat products? Don't those test as alkaline too? Everything you eat or drink will be formed into acid or alkaline chemical slush (called ash) during the process of digestion. A lime or lemon may be referred to as a natural citric acid, but once it is digested, it becomes alkaline. It's not the "before" ingestion, it's the "during" digestion that counts for your body. Citrus fruits, apple cider vinegar, and tomatoes are all considered very acidic but alkalize the body during digestion. Meat is the opposite. It will test alkaline before you eat it, but the process of digesting it acidifies it.

A short list of really common acid-forming foods is as follows: red meats; bread and wheat products; most grains, including corn, rye, oats, quinoa, and pastas; sugary beverages and snacks; all alcoholic drinks; fried foods; and most dairy products. You can see how the common, modern menu contributes to people having acid problems.

Chia seeds are moderately alkalizing! It's all that calcium they have; remember that chia has more calcium by weight than milk. And, unlike milk, chia doesn't process as an acid when you digest it.

Did you know that if your body isn't able to properly process the food you eat, this can also contribute to weight gain? Harmful amounts of yeast and fungus flourish in an acid environment. They make it harder for your body to absorb the nutrition it needs. The yeast can actually act like a type of parasite, eating nutrients you need. This can actually make you feel hungrier and crave sugar, which in turns feeds yeast and causes it to multiply. The cycle then repeats itself. An alkaline diet helps bring your body's pH into balance and flushes your system of yeast and fungi overgrowth.

Once you have decided to embrace a healthier lifestyle by eating fewer acid-forming foods, you may just wake up a little more cheerful and with a little less brain fog. Your body won't have to fight so hard to keep you in the "neutral zone" and it can go on to strengthen and win other battles to create better health. You will probably notice more energy, better memory, and less digestive problems.

These recipes focus on alkaline ingredients. You can make a surprising selection of tasty things to add to your menu when you keep alkaline ingredients in mind. Remember, mixing acid and alkaline ingredients isn't bad. There are many healthy foods that process as acids; it's important to not let the pH dictate everything you eat.

COOL CHIA CANTALOUPE SOUP

Do you have half a cantaloupe left over from making a fruit salad? If you do, that is extremely good news. Cantaloupes are a lovely, fragrant, alkaline food. This lovely, creamy soup just may be the highlight of your next supper! It is so densely rich in micronutrients and with the major component of low-fat yogurt, you will get a lovely dose of the good bacteria your body needs to digest. It is a snap to make ahead of time in your blender and can be your go-to soup when cantaloupes are in season.

INGREDIENTS:

 ½ of a very ripe cantaloupe, cut into manageable chunks
 1 cucumber, peeled and diced into manageable chunks
 ¾ cup low-fat yogurt
 2 limes, zested and juiced
 1 teaspoon ground cumin
 2 tablespoons agave nectar or honey
 1 tablespoon dry chia
 ¼ teaspoon cayenne pepper

INSTRUCTIONS:

In your blender place the cantaloupe chunks and blend. You may need to work in portions to accommodate the chunks. Once the cantaloupe has been pureed, add the cucumber pieces, yogurt, lime juice, and the seasonings. Blend until smooth. If the melon and cucumber were chilled, you can serve this cold soup right away. Just pour the puree into your soup bowls and you're ready to serve. This is really super when chilled! If your fruit wasn't refrigerated, just put the blender jar in the fridge until nice and chilled.

TROPICAL BREEZE COOL GREEN POPSICLE

Don't be afraid of this pop's super green color! It's delicious. You'll be amazed at the tropical fruity flavor of these popsicles! Banana, pineapple, spinach, lime, and chia seeds are all alkaline, and yogurt is neutral. These popsicles are creamy, fresh, and very fruity. If you close your eyes, you won't even notice there's spinach in them. These can be a cool solution for kids who hate leafy greens—they won't have a problem with them if they can't taste them at all!

INGREDIENTS:

 1 banana
 1 ½ cups pineapple chunks, drained

2 handfuls of fresh spinach
3 tablespoons plain yogurt
1 tablespoon nondairy creamer
1 teaspoon chia
1 lime, zested and juiced

INSTRUCTIONS:
In your mini chopper add the spinach and pineapple chunks. Pulse to chop thoroughly. Add the banana, yogurt, nondairy creamer, lime juice, and zest. Pulse to combine. Freeze so that when you need to take a "mini-vacation to Hawaii," you and your popsicle will be ready for take-off.

Note: This popsicle has one particularly amazing ingredient: the pineapple. Pineapple's most potent enzyme is bromelain. It's a digestive enzyme that helps you break down protein and fats. It also helps reduce inflammation. Try to get a fresh pineapple whenever you can to maximize the nutritional value (canned fruits are heated).

Pineapple also has manganese, vitamin C, vitamin B1 (thiamin), copper, fiber, and vitamin B6. Manganese is important because nutritionists say that it can boost your mood. Vitamin B6 helps you convert tryptophan into serotonin, which also helps your mood.

You might also be in a better mood if you had more energy. Look no further than the pineapple again! It's sweet, as you know, with the natural sugar fructose. Fructose is rich in carbohydrates, so it will break down quickly, giving you energy right away. However, the pineapple also has fiber (along with the chia seeds), which slows down the conversion of carbohydrates into sugars to provide lasting energy as well. Manganese not only boosts your mood; it, along with thiamin, is essential to metabolizing the carbohydrates in the pineapple and giving you more energy.

General Tips and Tricks for Better Health

There are a few general tips and tricks you can easily use for better overall health. They're not all 100 percent chia seed–related, but they're too valuable to ignore. There are small, surprisingly easy changes or activities you can undertake that will make the advice in this book work much better.

First, reality check: Are you willing to make small, positive changes that will dramatically change your life? Will you add a few small changes that will add up to a happier *you*? We're not all going to be supermodels (who would want to?), sports idols, or famous celebrities. There are some things you just can't control, like heredity. Your heredity plays an important role in your body shape, size, and build. Don't lament! Work with what you have and start re-creating the best *you*. Don't let other people tell you how you "should" look. A look isn't nearly as important as good health. A lot of the role models you see in advertisements, movies, and magazines have been edited, anyway. They don't actually look like what you see, so you can't aspire to be something that doesn't exist.

Second, attitude adjustment: Choose to be happy. Don't waste your brain power on negative thoughts, such as, "I'll be happy when I lose XXX pounds, my joints don't hurt, my stomach problems lessen, or I have more energy." Start being happy now! Everyone can find at least one thing that he or she is grateful for. When you focus on what is actually going right in your life, you'll notice more of the same. Instead of saying, "I'll be happy when...", say, "I am so rich because . . ." This phrase forces your mind to come up with reasons why you might be rich. Do you have a safe house? Do you have good health? Do you have a pet who loves you? These are all reasons someone could consider themselves wealthy. Your health is your wealth, and you can always improve your health!

Third, be your own cheerleader: Compliment yourself for a job well done. Praise yourself for keeping a positive attitude, even when the world around you seems more than a little chaotic. Once you learn to rid yourself of any streaming negative thoughts, you will notice that you feel better about yourself. It's great! Focus on what went right during the day. Focus not on fighting "reality" but on accepting what is and what you cannot control. Be good to you by not playing the "blame game." Take responsibility for your life, both good and bad. Please remember that no one sees the world as you do. There are several ways to view a situation and there could be several positive ways to handle it. Your way may not always work for everyone.

When making changes in your lifestyle, such as adding exercise or eating differently, it's important for *you* to be on your own side. If you're too harsh about the changes (e.g., getting really upset if it rains when you wanted to go for a walk, or becoming aggravated if you're tempted into having a sweet one day), you build up a negative environment inside your mind that's not conductive to sticking with, and having fun with, your new, healthier way of living.

Fourth, good nutrition, exercise, and use of free time: We cannot say enough about good, sound food choices. Let the greengrocer be your pharmacy. The foods you put into your body are its fuel. Your body will tell you how much better it feels once you start feeding it all the micronutrients and macronutrients it requires.

You have to move it! Everyone has twenty-four hours in a day, however, spending two hours at the gym doesn't work for most people. You must make a small change to include a little exercise. Whether it is just a brisk walk around the block a couple of times, shooting hoops with the kids, taking tango lessons, or doing a little yoga, you must move your body. Choose what works for you, but move it.

Save a little *me* time. You deserve it! What do you truly enjoy? Twenty minutes of solitude? Twenty minutes of reading? Twenty minutes of chatting with friends? Twenty minutes of . . .? It's important to relax. Twenty-four hours—that's what we get. You can spare twenty minutes for *you*. When you take good care of yourself first, you're ready to take care of all the issues and people in your life. Don't neglect yourself and your own mental well-being. Banish all "if onlys" and all regrets. That was in the past. You're looking forward to the future!

GO TO THE GROCERY FOR YOUR HEALTH

When you or any of your friends went to the doctor for your last few check-ups, did the doctor ask, "Generally, what are you eating as typical breakfasts, lunches, and dinners?"

No? We got the same response. "No." Blood pressure too high? Cholesterol too high? Feel tired all the time? They want to know about your ailments, not what you are doing to actively prevent things from going wrong with your health. They want to say, "Here is a pill to help correct that." Pharmaceutical companies offer "zillions" of dollars to medical schools and research programs. Medical schools rarely focus on nutrition, diet, and preventive health techniques.

Dr. Joseph Mercola, the physician and author, states,[47] "Modern humans are facing a slew of 'modern' diseases and conditions that simply weren't seen—or were only rarely seen—in ancient times. Cancer, heart disease, diabetes, obesity—all of these would apply. Quite simply, we've strayed too far from the foods we are designed to

---

47   Dr. Joseph Mercola, "When Fire Met Food: The Brains of Early Humans Grew Bigger," http://articles.mercola.com/sites/articles/archive/2012/11/10/cooked-food-diet.aspx (Accessed 22 October 2013)

eat, so going back to basics and refocusing your diet on fresh, whole, unprocessed, 'real' food can improve just about anyone's health."

Plants contain not only vitamins and minerals and fiber but also special plant compounds with healing properties called phytonutrients (or phytochemicals). *Phytochemicals* are medicinal molecules, such as curcumin in turmeric, glucosinolate in broccoli, anthocyanidins in berries and black rice, and so on. Different phytonutrients have different properties. Some provide natural detoxification. Each is important in its own way and when eaten together in the right proportion, they can have a dramatic effect on your health.

Dr. Mark Hyman states, "We all have hundreds of thousands of little energy factories called mitochondria in our cells, which are our energy factories. They manufacture ATP, which is our energy fuel. Provide your energy factories with a nutrient-dense diet and some exercise and watch how your body responds."

He also states, "Quality foods drive our gene function, metabolism, and health. It is not simply a matter of your weight, or calories in/calories out. Eating powerful, gene-altering, whole, real, fresh food that you cook yourself can rapidly change your biology. You will lose weight by getting your systems in balance, not by starving yourself."[48]

FIGHT INFLAMMATION

Inflammation is part of the body's immune response. It is the swelling, reddened, heated, and pain-produced state of the body as a reaction to injury or infection. Inflammation is how the body heals itself by focusing more nourishment and immune activity on the required area.

---

48   Dr. Mark Hyman, "How to Give Yourself a Metabolic Tune-Up," *Huffington Post*, http://www.huffingtonpost.com/dr-mark-hyman/how-to-give-yourself-a-me_b_506431.html (Accessed 22 October 2013)

However, sometimes the inflammatory process goes wrong. Wrong inflammatory responses can include allergies (overreacting to a harmless substance such as pollen), overreactions to minor injuries, overreacting to certain common foods or food additives, and much more. Sometimes, you don't notice inflammation at all. If an internal organ doesn't hurt but has a low-grade inflammation, you won't feel it at all.

Sometimes inflammation can cause further inflammation. These conditions cause self-perpetuating inflammation, which is bad for you. Genetics, stress, and exposure to environmental toxins all have bearing on a person's level of persistent, low-level inflammation throughout his or her body. This condition increases the risk of major health problems and disease. Highly processed foods, chemical additives, preservatives, hydrogenated oils, and other modern food modifications can all cause low-level inflammation. You might not feel it, but it can increase the risk of health problems. Natural foods provide the nutrients your body needs to fight the inflammatory effects.

According the Franklin Institute, trans fats are particularly detrimental to the health of the brain.[49] So put down that doughnut or french fry and save your brain too!

BEAT THE AFTERNOON SLUMP

You've been getting through your to-do list and then, all of a sudden, *bam*! You run into a brick wall called the afternoon slump. It hits after lunch around 2:00 PM—the dreaded circadian trough. It can be a sugar slump, as insulin clears away the sugars you may have consumed at lunch. This is a time when people reach for another sweet snack, or a cup of coffee. Caffeine and sugar aren't a great long-term answer for the slump.

---

49 Franklin Institute, "Nourishment–Fats," http://www.fi.edu/learn/brain/fats.html (Accessed 20 October 2013)

You already know about how chia can help balance blood sugar and slow the conversion of carbs into sugars. This works at lunch time too and you may be able to avoid the slump. There are other ways to fight the slump as well! Try taking a brisk walk outdoors. Deeply breathe the fresh outdoor air. Can't get outside? You can do breathing exercises in your chair. Try walking over to a fellow associate for a quick question instead of emailing or calling. Try having a tiny snack of protein enhanced with chia to boost your energy. An ice-cold beverage with chia seeds can also wake you up.

BE CAREFUL OF BEING OBSESSED WITH ORGANIC

Don't get confused about organic foods; this label just means how it was grown. Some fruits and veggies are better bought organic if they have thin or no skins where pesticides most likely were sprayed. However, if you purchase an "organic meal" with cheese sauce and pasta that is high in calories and loaded with sugars, well, that may not have harmful chemicals, but it's still not good for you. Too much sugar—even if it's organic and non-GMO—isn't good for your health. Know what you are putting in your body with a combination of organic foods and wise choices.

BE CAREFUL WHEN CONSUMING ALCOHOL

If you choose to drink alcoholic drinks, beware of the calories. An ounce of alcohol contains the number of calories equivalent to those in a baked potato or a glass of milk! It's more than you'd think! Along with a few "nibbles" before dinner and a drink or two, *wow*, you have consumed a lot of calories even before dinner—and you still don't feel full at all. A ten-ounce margarita can have up to 550 calories. Because it's just a drink, people don't notice. A couple of drinks with all those empty calories with no nutritional benefit can add up to a whole day's worth of calories!

We are just saying you should be thoughtful. Adding all those calories and the damage any alcohol does to organs may not be worth it. If you want to be a part of the party, just ask for club soda with a twist of lime or lemon or a small glass of red wine—you won't be singled out, and it's a healthier choice.

SAY "NO, THANKS" TO DESSERT

People will assume you are watching your weight if you say no to dessert. But it is not a case of being "good" or "bad"—if you are full, stop eating. If you are still hungry, have a little dessert so that you don't feel deprived. People who feel deprived or "punished" by not having dessert can overeat later on or give in to dessert-related cravings. If you have a small portion of dessert, you won't feel left out or deprived. People come in all shapes and sizes. We are wishing you physical and emotional well-being. Don't stress! Just be thoughtful.

HAVE A PLAN B

A well-stocked pantry can be your go-to meal when time is short or plans abruptly change. It is wise to have a plan B so that you don't think, "Oh, I'll just pick up fast food on the way home." Your plan B should be fast, easy, truly healthy, and something everyone likes. If the family says, "Let's just pick up something," you can say, "Let's keep it simple. We have plan B, and everyone likes our plan B." You will save a lot of money and crankiness this way.

FLOSS, FLOSS, FLOSS

Because you will be consuming more veggies and tiny seeds from fruits and chia, it is important that you floss before bed. If you don't floss, your gums become inflamed, which makes it easier for the bad bacteria to enter your bloodstream. When that nasty bacteria enters your bloodstream, it can cause inflammation all over your body. Some studies show that bad bacteria from the mouth can influence heart disease. It's serious business, but the mouth is easy enough to keep clean with regular brushing and flossing. Internal inflammation is your enemy, and you can fight it with floss.

GET VITAMIN SUNSHINE

Researchers estimate that only a small percentage of middle-age Americans get enough vitamin D through their diet or sunshine exposure. It is recommended that everyone get outside to expose (at least) their faces and hands to the sun for fifteen minutes per day with no sunscreen. "Our skin contains provitamin D3 which interacts with ultraviolet-B to produce vitamin D3. The liver and kidneys also contribute to further synthesizing the exact vitamin D the body needs," states *American Journal of Clinical Nutrition*.[50]

Fifteen minutes is not enough to get a tan, dry out the skin, become wrinkly, or drastically increase the risk of skin cancer. However, if you have a darker skin pigmentation, or if you live at a very northern latitude, the sun might not be strong enough to produce enough vitamin D. You might want to take a supplement as well and make sure you get your vitamin D3 levels tested by your doctor. So step away from your electronic screens and try to get outside more!

UP YOUR STAMINA

By engaging in low-intensity exercise for twenty minutes per day, three to four times per week, you will reduce that rundown feeling by 65 percent and boost your energy levels by 20 percent,

---

50   Michael F. Holick, "Sunlight and Vitamin D for Bone Health and Prevention of Autoimmune Diseases, Cancers, and Cardiovascular Disease," *American Journal of Clinical Nutrition*, http://ajcn.nutrition.org/content/80/6/1678S.full (Accessed 22 October 2013)

studies show.[51] Just by taking a brisk walk with the dog, dancing in your living room, or playing tag with the kids, you can trigger the release of dopamine in your brain. This lovely, feel-good chemical makes you feel more vigorous.

PRACTICE WILLPOWER

According to a Ian Newby Clarke, a psychologist at Gulph, it can take a varying amount of time for each person to get comfortable with some of the healthy changes you'd like to make to your lifestyle.[52] It is practice, practice, practice! Making a little change is like exercise, and it becomes easier with time. Build up slowly so that you don't freak out and go back to the the way it was. We bet you won't even want to. Habits are formed by doing little bits each day. Rome wasn't built in a day and neither is a healthier lifestyle. Remind yourself daily of the rewards (are you going for more energy?) and pay attention to your experiences (savor a bite of dark chocolate), so that you're focusing on the positive.

Hit with a craving? Have a bite of the item you want. If you feel deprived, you're more likely to break down and overdo it later. Having a bite or two is not going to ruin your new health efforts. Cravings are also quieted by eating a larger variety of foods in general. You may not even need any willpower to resist a craving that's no longer occurring for you.

MANAGE AGING METABOLISMS

Ladies over forty years of age have to wrestle with their changing hormones, stress, empty nest syndrome, aging parents, the list

---

51   CBC News, "Low-Intensity Exercise Can Boost Energy, Curb Fatigue: Study," http://www.cbc.ca/news/technology/low-intensity-exercise-can-boost-energy-curb-fatigue-study-1.714677 (Accessed 22 October 2013)

52   Ian Newby-Clarke, "Creatures Of Habit: How Long?", *Psychology Today*, http://www.psychologytoday.com/blog/creatures-habit/200912/how-long (Accessed 21 October 2013)

goes on and on. Your metabolism slows down with age, and it is easy to gain a pound per year if you don't watch out.

Researchers at the University of Virginia found that power-walking (walking as fast as you can) for shorter distances will burn five times more abdominal fat than taking a stroll for longer distances, even if the same number of calories are burned. This works for anyone, both men and women.

DO NOT STARVE YOURSELF!

When you eat less than your body's biological needs (about 1,200 calories for most people), your body's metabolism kicks into starvation mode. This makes the body want to store fat even more than usual. The body will then ferociously try to hang onto any fat as you can't tell your body that this isn't a famine. For self-preservation it will start breaking down muscle tissue for energy along with fat tissue. This slows your whole metabolism. Not good! If weight loss is a goal for you, eat enough so that you feel full at meals, and have a small, nutritious snack every three to four hours to keep yourself from going on a feeding frenzy later in the evening or triggering the body's starvation responses.

FEED YOUR SKIN

"Chia seeds contain omega-3 oils, which have been used to treat a number of skin disorders," explains Dr. Oscar Hevia, a cosmetic dermatologist and founder of the Hevia Center for Research. "Omega-3 oil can potentially provide a number of beneficial effects for the skin, including protection of the top skin layer and promotion of wound healing, among others."[53]

---

53 Stephanie Nolasco, "Can Chia Seeds Really Fight Wrinkles? Experts Weigh In," *Fox News Magazine*, http://magazine.foxnews.com/style-beauty/can-chia-seeds-really-fight-wrinkles-experts-weigh (Accessed 21 October 2013)

GET YOUR PROTEIN

You have read in this book about chia being a complete protein. A new study in the *American Journal of Clinical Nutrition* reported that omega-3s may also stimulate muscle protein synthesis in older adults.[54] Good news, as many older adults just don't get enough protein in their eating habits.

FEED YOUR BRAIN

According to the Franklin Institute, "trans fats are particularly detrimental for the health of the brain. Trans fats imitate healthy fats and disrupt neurological activity due to the abnormal shape and lack of flexibility."[55] Keep to the healthy fats such as—you guessed it—omega-3s.

TAKE CARE WHEN EATING OUT

Eating out is the danger zone if you let it be one! Watch out for falling bread sticks, chips and salsa, and biscuits that are offered "complimentary" at restaurants before your meal arrives. This is a bumpy road! All of the above add a load of calories and have no real nutrient value. You already know which restaurants come in high on the calorie count scale with the "cheddar/bacon/whammie burger" or the "crispy chicken soaked in fat sauce."

Restaurants want their portions to look generous so that everyone will think that it's a good value. Look out for huge plates

---

54 Gordon I Smith, Philip Atherton, Dominic N Reeds, B Selma Mohammed, Debbie Rankin, Michael J Rennie, and Bettina Mittendorfer, "Dietary Omega-3 Fatty Acid Supplementation Increases the Rate of Muscle Protein Synthesis in Older Adults: A Randomized Controlled Trial," *American Journal of Clinical Nutrition*, http://ajcn.nutrition.org/content/early/2010/12/15/ajcn.110.005611 (Accessed 21 October 2013)
55 Franklin Institute, "Nourishment–Fats," http://www.fi.edu/learn/brain/fats.html (Accessed 20 October 2013)

and giant piles of food. Remember that it's OK to get a doggy box or a to-go cup and stop eating when you feel full. Belonging to the "clean plate club" is no longer the goal. You should still enjoy restaurants, but know the ins and outs of what's best to order and remember to avoid the pitfalls such as huge plates and loads of breadsticks.

TAKE ADVANTAGE OF NATURAL ANTIBIOTICS

Lime juice, garlic, and yogurt are some of Mother Nature's natural antibiotics and antifungal agents. Lime juice, strawberries, and broccoli all have quantities of vitamin C, which strengthens the immune system, and they're acidic enough to kill some types of bacteria. Garlic contains quantities of allicin, which will kill some of the bad bacteria. Mustard can also kill some strains of harmful bacteria. Yogurt contains the good bacteria, which crowds out the bad guys. Keep Mother Nature on your team.

AVOID EATING TOO QUICKLY AND TOO LATE

It takes twenty minutes for your tummy to tell your brain it has had enough food. The stomach signals the brain with chemicals, not through nerves, that's why it's so slow. The *Journal of American Dietetic Association* found that slow eaters took in fewer calories and felt like they had eaten more.[56] Just like pennies add up a little at a time, so do calories, especially calories that don't provide all the nutrients your body requires.

If your body is too busy processing a full stomach just before bed, it has no time to burn fat while you sleep. Wow! Burn

---

56 Emily Creasy, *MS, RD, LD*, "What Is True About Eating Slower to Promote Weight Loss?" *Nutrition Remarks*, http://www.nutritionremarks. com/2012/02/14/eating-slower-to-promote-weight-loss/ (Accessed 20 October 2013)

calories while you sleep?! Studies have shown that completing dinner a couple of hours before your bedtime provides your body with a head start. Your liver will use up all the glycogen in your body to regulate your blood sugar levels. When that task is complete, it moves onto body fat! We aim to have completed dinner at least two to three hours before bed.

If dinner seems like a long-past memory, try chewing a piece of sugarless gum. Hydrate your body with a little chia fresca, deeply breathe for five minutes, have a cup of caffeine-free tea, or just brush your teeth again. The craving will pass, and you will sleep more soundly.

TAKE CARE WITH CHOLESTEROL MEDS

Some people will say, "I take cholesterol medicine, therefore I don't need to be so careful about what I eat." *Wrong!* This medication works best when it is combined with a healthy eating style. Remember that your goal is to get off these medications (if possible) so that they don't harm your liver over time. Medication does not have to be inevitable. If you have to be on cholesterol medication, you should likely also be supplementing with coenzyme Q10, as this medication type is known for removing this heart-essential nutrient from the body. Be sure to ask your doctor whether any of your medications are "drug muggers" and whether you should be supplementing to counteract any mugging effects. There may be a time in the near future when you walk into your doctor's office and the doctor will be examining a better you!

DECIDE WHETHER TO COOK IT OR NOT TO COOK IT

It seems it is a win-some/lose-some proposition. The red pigment in tomatoes becomes more concentrated by cooking, but you lose amounts of vitamins C and B. The same applies to blueberries.

The anthocyanins in the blue pigment increase during cooking, but vitamins C and B are lost. Broccoli is another case where if cooked it loses the enzyme myrosinase, which coverts sulforaphane to its cancer-fighting active form but when eaten raw it has as much vitamin C and fiber as an orange. Raw broccoli has vitamin A, potassium, and extra protein. We say vary the way you consume, in terms of being cooked or not cooked.

Some foods are just better off uncooked completely. These include spinach leaves, most fruits, and cabbage. Other foods such as broccoli tend to expel their nutrients when heated. That's why you'll see steaming broccoli as a recommendation here, if you have to cook it at all. For instance, if broccoli is cooked in water, it will expel the nutrients into the water, which is then generally poured off. If, however, you're making a soup, for instance, and you intend to consume the water a veggie was cooked in, you'll still get the nutrients.

Canned goods *are* cooked! That can of pineapple, jug of juice, or can of soup has been cooked, and likely at quite a high temperature. Juice and canned fruit need to be pasteurized to give them the shelf life stores require for safety. In the case of canned soups, most of the nutrients in the vegetables have likely been cooked out by the time you eat the soup. Whenever you can, select fresh fruits and make soups at home so that you'll know exactly how the food was prepared.

Canned soup is convenient, but it is often high in sodium. (Yes, you can get low-sodium versions, but that limits your selection of flavors and brands.) You already know about cooking out nutrients, but remember that many cans are lined with the chemical BPA, which has been linked to infertility, heart disease, weight gain, and diabetes. Studies have shown that it's a type of estrogen mimic in the human body, so it can unbalance your hormones.

So, instead of forgoing soup altogether, get out your soup pot and get cooking. Most soups freeze well, so if you like the convenience or portion control of "almost instant" soup, freeze your homemade soup in individual serving containers that seal tightly against freezer burn. Soup doesn't have to take all day to cook! Just look at some of the soup recipes in this book—they're fast and easy! There's more out there too; with the Internet at your fingertips, you can find many tasty recipes that cook in thirty minutes or less.

PLATE IN THE KITCHEN

If you plate in the kitchen, there is a likelihood that you and your family will eat less than you would when serving buffet-style. When people are just thinking about another helping, it appears that people hesitate to go back to the kitchen for more. Also, keep in mind your plate size. A large plate (no matter who is filling it) will tend to be piled with more food and also tempt people to eat more. Measure your plates and choose a medium size. You might be surprised at the visual effect.

AIM FOR ONE POUND PER WEEK

If you feel you're on the heavier side of where you would like to be, weight-wise, consider this: losing one pound per week should be your goal. We bet you've seen magazine articles that claim, "I lost thirteen pounds in one week! See how I did it!" Well, that's not realistic, and it's hard on your body. Your body could go into starvation mode and make it even harder to lose weight. A healthy eating style encourages you and your body to be satisfied so that you will continue to eat healthily for the rest of your life; food isn't supposed to be a constant battle between what tastes good and what *is* good for you.

Did you know that one pound of fat is equal to about 3,500 calories? So, if you eliminated one sugar-laden soft drink and one bagel per day for one week—ta-da! That would be one pound. Skipping a super-sweet coffee drink (e.g., a latte) or a white-flour breakfast treat item each day isn't a big deal. It's a small change to go from a latte to a tasty smoothie. Making a change doesn't have to be a big deal because each little bit adds up. Each pound you lose lessens the stress on your joints, knees, and lower back. Add a couple of cool glasses of chia fresca (with either lime or lemon) to keep yourself feeling hydrated and keep the fullness factor. As you now know, adding that lime or lemon to water will boost your alkaline intake and make your body smile.

TAKE CARE WITH VITAMIN AND MINERAL SUPPLEMENTS

Because of overfarming and food packaging, we are not receiving the vitamins and nutrients our grandparents received for the same produce we buy today. You may feel you would like to at least take a multivitamin with minerals to fill in any gaps in your eating habits (or in plants that were grown on overfarmed land).

Be sure to do your research on supplement brands and content. You don't have to spend a bundle or buy the most expensive supplements out there. Vitamin D3, for example, can be had for pennies a day. There's a lot of "fluff" out there masquerading as essential nutrition boosters. Watch out for fillers such as harmless starches or binders. Look for the amount of vitamins or minerals contained in each serving. (Is a serving one, two, or more pills per day?) Some forms of some nutrients work better for some people than they do for others. Is the calcium that works best for you calcium citrate or calcium carbonate or calcium gluconate? You may have to try a few brands or a few sources (oyster shell, bone meal, dairy-derived) to find the one that works best for you.

Be sure to avoid overload. Do you actually *need* a multivitamin with iron in it? Some people's diet naturally contains enough iron that if they took a supplement with iron, it would be too much. Too much iron oxidizes and can cause inflammation. You can always get tested to see what you're short of and what you may need to add more of.

Remember that your doctor is your helper. If you suspect that you're deficient in any type of vitamin or mineral, ask to get tested. Doctors won't offer tests just offhand (most of the time); you've got to do the research and then ask for the test.

AVOID BEING TOO CORN-Y

Did you know that corn is not a vegetable? It is actually a grain! It is served and treated as a veggie, but there are actually little pockets of starch and sugar on that cob. You may want to think about your plate when you see this grain looking pretty, as it's not as good for you as a vegetable. Corn does have carotenoids and fiber, but you have to eat a lot of it while it's fresh to get the most of these benefits. Also keep in mind the genetic modification of many types of corn. Most modified corn has been altered so that it will resist weeds, resist pesticides, kill pests, keep for longer periods of time, look fresher, and grow faster. Notice that "be healthier" and "contain more nutrients" or even "taste better" are not on the list of modifications. You can enjoy corn and corn snacks in moderation, but do keep in mind that corn is a grain and should be treated like one.

WATCH SERVING SIZE WHEN LABEL READING

OK, you've got it. Read the labels of foods before you buy them. But don't glaze over the "portion" section, as it can be easy to miss. The calorie count on the package is *only* for the serving size the package states. Is the serving size ridiculously small? Is it just one cookie, when most people eat two or three? Really! That can be a huge difference and may require a little math on your part. Some products will claim a super-low calorie count on the front, but, then, when you look at the serving size, of course the count is low but you can barely eat any of the product to make up the one serving that had the advertised calories.

CHEW GUM

We have read that chewing gum stimulates the salivary glands and may aid in washing away accumulated acid in the gut. Keeping fresh saliva flowing over the teeth and gums also promotes a healthy mouth. Chewing sugar-free gum also promotes fresher breath. Sometimes we also use sugar-free gum to have that "little sweet" after dinner while waiting for our brains to catch up and send the full signal.

Gums with sugar-free sweeteners such as stevia or xylitol may also help kill cavity-causing bacteria while you chew them. If snacking is your problem, a sugar-free gum can help. It keeps the mouth busy with chewing and your brain entertained with its sweetness. Find a sugar-free flavor that you really enjoy and give chewing gum a try.

Introduction to General and Fun Recipes

The MySeeds Test Kitchen understands that *life* happens. We are not health *zealots*—just proponents! We do eat white flour (sometimes), and we do put real whipped cream on a special dessert (sometimes). We do eat a small piece of birthday cake. We do eat pizza out with friends. Oh, my gosh, we have cravings for a hamburger—*so what*? Once in a while works fine for us. We know that our bodies will swing back to the "sweet spot." Eating anything occasionally is not going to hurt you. Feeling severely deprived can be the cause of eating a whole bag of chips or sticking your face in the ice cream. Don't go there!

We take a commonsense approach to food and what we have read over the years. Lightly cooked or raw veggies, fruits, beans, a few whole grains, lean protein, not very much dairy, and a sprinkle of chia here and there—it is *all* good.

You will notice that there are no nutrition facts or calorie counts on any of the recipes in this book. We feel that if you know you are eating in a healthy manner, all that weighing, counting, and so forth takes some of the joy out of having a nice, fresh, pretty meal. Once you get the hang of perhaps eating a bit more body-friendly, you won't want to add more *stress* to your life. Everyone's body metabolism is different. How you burn calories will be different from how your friends or other family members do. That's OK! Just find what works for you.

Your family may balk at a life change (e.g., the introduction of a meatless night). You may want to become ninja-like. Ask your family to help plan the week's meals so that the weekly grocery shopping is pre-established and the kitchen is fully stocked. It is just plain sad that so many children don't know how to prepare a meal or what constitutes a balanced diet. Many children can't even identify a variety of vegetables, let alone know what to do with them. Eating together, cooking together, and laughing together should be the family's goal—even if it is not every day because of overly busy schedules. Practice, practice, and more practice will let this become routine.

The following recipes can be a starting platform for you. If your family doesn't like an ingredient, substitute. You will notice that there are no Brussels sprouts in *any* of our recipes. The reason? We don't like them, but they are good for you. So what? Not everyone is going to like everything, but you need to try before you make up your mind. Kids generally need to be exposed six to eight times to something new before it is accepted as eatable. If you're cooking for kids, be sure to see the section on picky eaters in this book for some great tips.

The recipes in this section are focused on fun and variety. There's nothing boring or bland in here. You *will* find a few sweets too. If you want something sweet, it's better to have a bite of portion-controlled real sugar than it is to deprive yourself or resort to unhealthy artificial sweeteners. Both deprivation and chemicals can lead to a really unhealthy desire to overeat later on. Some of these recipes also illustrate points such as gluten-free foods, saving money on gourmet foods, or making low-sugar recipes with chia.

KNIFE AND FORK CHIA PIZZA

We have a fast and easy dip that we are just crazy about. With chopped frozen spinach, some cheeses, and shredded chicken, what could be better? Well, if you put this dip on a readymade personal pizza round and top it with a little salad and marinated mushrooms, you have the answer! Healthy and *awesome*!

If you would like the pizza to be nearly instant, you can make up the dip and mushrooms earlier (even a day or two when stored in the fridge) and put the pizza together in as much time as it takes for the oven to heat. The dip will coat about three personal pizzas.

INGREDIENTS:
FOR THE DIP:
    1 10-ounce box of chopped spinach
    1 precooked chicken breast (shredded)
    2 tablespoons onion
    3 ounces cream cheese
    ½ cup Swiss cheese (shredded)
    2 tablespoons low-fat plain yogurt
    2 tablespoons chia gel

¼ teaspoon nutmeg

1 small sweet red pepper, deseeded and chopped

1 pinch red pepper flakes

FOR THE PIZZA BREAD & GREENS TOPPING

3 pre-made personal size pizza bread rounds

1 handful torn salad greens of choice

1 average sized tomato (diced)

¼ inch round of a red onion (diced)

FOR THE MUSHROOMS:

1 pound cleaned, sliced mushrooms

¼ cup red wine vinegar

¼ cup olive oil

⅛ cup chopped onion

2 cloves minced garlic

1 teaspoon dry mustard

1 tablespoon agave or honey

INSTRUCTIONS:

FOR THE DIP:

Microwave the block of spinach in a covered dish for about four minutes on high. Use a fork to squeeze out the water. In the same dish, add the cooked, shredded chicken, and all the other ingredients. Re-cover and microwave for about two minutes. Stir to combine. (Chill if not using soon and then warm it back up in the microwave when ready to make the pizza.)

FOR THE MUSHROOMS:

In a medium saucepan, mix all the ingredients together and then add the mushrooms. Simmer for about ten minutes while stirring occasionally. (Chill if not using soon.)

Coat the pizza rounds evenly with the spinach dip. Bake per the instructions of your packaging, which is usually about eight minutes.

In a bowl place your salad greens (e.g., spinach, arugula, torn red leaf lettuce), thin slivers of red onion, and diced tomato. Drain the mushrooms. Assemble the salad on top of the freshly baked crusts and top with the mushrooms. Yeah! Pizza night!

CITRUS CHIA CHIFFON DESSERT

Whether you choose lime or lemon for this dessert, you are going to be preparing a truly delightful experience. We make ours in an eight-and-a-half-inch springform pan but you can also use an eight- or nine-inch pie pan. The crust is low in fat and clings together nicely, thanks to the chia gel, and doesn't get soggy. The chiffon mousse is light and zippy. Although it is a little time-consuming to make, this recipe is well worth the effort and must be made ahead of time, as it must chill for about two hours before you serve. You will want to have at least four limes or lemons to get the zest and juice needed. This recipe makes eight servings.

INGREDIENTS:
FOR THE SIMPLE SYRUP:
  1 cup water
  ½ cup sugar
  2 tablespoons lemon or lime zest

FOR THE CRUST:
  1 cup graham cracker crumbs (about 6–8 crackers)
  ¼ cup macadamia nuts or pecans
  2 tablespoons white chocolate chips
  Zest of one lime or lemon (to match the filling)
  1 tablespoon brown sugar
  2 tablespoons melted butter
  1 tablespoon chia gel

For the mousse:

    1 envelope unflavored gelatin

    ½ cup sugar (will be divided)

    2 eggs, separated (place the whites in a large bowl to be beaten)

    ⅓ cup fresh lime or lemon juice (to match the crust)

    1 cup whipping cream (or 2 cups premade whipped topping)

    1 teaspoon vanilla

INSTRUCTIONS:

For the simple syrup:

In a saucepan simmer the water, sugar, and zest for about half an hour, stirring occasionally. Once the simple syrup has cooled to just warm, strain the zest from the syrup and then add it back into one-third cup of your syrup. Discard the remaining syrup.

    While the syrup is simmering, you can make the crust.

For the crust:

In your mini chopper crumble the graham crackers. Pour into a small bowl. Follow with the nuts, chopping them and then adding them to the bowl. Next chop the chocolate chips and add them to the bowl. Add the zest, brown sugar, melted butter, and chia gel. Stir to combine while breaking up any clumps and any large pieces of cracker or nut that were not chopped. Coat your pan of choice with cooking spray and press the crumbs onto the bottom (and sides if using a pie pan). Bake at 350 degrees Fahrenheit for eight to ten minutes. Cool.

For the mousse:

In the saucepan with the one-third cup syrup and zest, sprinkle the gelatin over the top of the syrup. Let stand for about a minute. Stir in the two egg yolks, lime juice, and one-quarter cup of sugar. Stir or whisk over low heat for about five minutes, until the mixture becomes frothy and thickens (but it will not be thick). Set aside to cool to room temperature.

Beat with your mixer the egg whites with two tablespoons of sugar until stiff.

In another bowl beat the whipping cream, the vanilla, and the last two tablespoons of sugar until thick. Fold in the egg whites while drizzling the citrus syrup over the mixture. When the mixture has incorporated, pour it into your prepared crust. Chill for several hours.

Note: As you may have noticed, we choose to use real whipping cream. We much prefer it over a faux whip cream. Wikipedia has the ingredients for premade whipped topping products, which are water, corn syrup and high fructose corn syrup, hydrogenated coconut and palm kernel oil, sodium caseinate, vanilla extract, xanthan and guar gums, polysorbate 60, and beta-carotene (for coloring).

CHIA BROWNIE BRITTLE

A friend of ours brought us a package of brownie bark from a specialty grocery store as a gift one holiday season. We said, "Oh, really! Delish! We *need* to make this." You'll save money when you make this expensive gourmet item in your own home. Impress your guests at any time of the year by serving a few pieces of this thin, crisp brittle. If Christmas is just around the corner, oftentimes after a fabulous meal, you are just too full to want a heavy dessert. But, well, chocolate puts the meal over the top. Just a little and you are satisfied.

Brownie brittle is easy to make and can obviously be made ahead of time to leave you the extra time you need to pull your holiday feast together.

INGREDIENTS:

2 large egg whites

½ cup granulated sugar

1 ½ tablespoons dark unsweetened cocoa powder

2 tablespoons vegetable oil

2 tablespoons chia gel

¼ teaspoon baking powder, rounded

¼ teaspoon vanilla

½ cup flour, sifted

½ chocolate dark mini chips or regular size chocolate chips

INSTRUCTIONS:

Preheat the oven to 325 degrees Fahrenheit and line a small-sided baking sheet (about 10 × 13 inches) with foil. The foil is a *must*! You will be peeling it off when the brittle has cooled.

In a mixing bowl whisk the egg whites until a little foamy. Keep whisking the whites and gradually add the sugar, cocoa powder, oil, chia gel, and vanilla. Next, whisk in the sifted flour, baking powder, and then the chocolate chips.

Pour the mixture in the center of the prepared baking sheet and spread the batter until it is as thin as possible. If need be, put in a few chips where there is batter only.

Bake for approximately twenty-five minutes. Look for cracking on the top and a dry appearance. Remove the pan and give the top of the brittle a tap with the back of a spoon. If the batter was a little thicker in some places, you may need to bake a little longer. Once the brittle has cooled, remove the foil and break or tear your chocolaty goodness into the size shards you would prefer.

SPICED-UP VEGGIE SPAGHETTI AND MEATBALLS

This spaghetti and meatball dinner is fast and will certainly tickle your taste buds! Fresh veggies lightly warmed in the chunky sauce will make this quick dinner an easy plan B if you come home late from work. This isn't your traditional, boring, jar spaghetti sauce that you've had a hundred times. Get out your spaghetti pot and start boiling the pasta! This serves about three people, or lunch is ready for tomorrow.

INGREDIENTS:

FOR THE MEATBALLS:

    1 pound ground turkey
    1 tablespoon dry chia
    4 tablespoons panko bread crumbs
    1 tablespoon chili powder
    1 garlic clove, smashed and diced
    ½ teaspoon ground cumin

FOR THE SAUCE:

    1 15-ounce can chunky tomatoes
    1 tablespoon dry chia (to thicken the sauce)
    ½ 4.5-ounce can of mild green chilies
    1 dash ground cloves
    ¼ teaspoon smoked paprika
    1 teaspoon ground cumin
    2 ½ tablespoons apple cider vinegar
    1 tablespoon molasses or dark brown sugar
    About 6 oz. pasta of choice (linguine)
    Large handful of broccoli florets
    1 large carrot, diagonal-cut into rounds
    Handful of mushrooms

INSTRUCTIONS:

To make the meatballs, just place the ground turkey, dry chia, chili powder, garlic, and panko crumbs into a bowl and combine by hand. Roll into about sixteen balls all approximately the same size, about one and one-half inches in diameter.

Start your water boiling for the pasta and follow the directions for cooking on the package. (It should be about twelve minutes.)

Next, bring out your large skillet and coat with cooking spray. Over medium-high heat brown the meatballs on all sides. Once browned, pour in the tomatoes, the chilies, and the remaining spices and chia. Cover, lower the heat, and simmer for about five minutes. Uncover and stir in the veggies to coat for about a minute or two. The spaghetti should be ready, and you can drain and serve.

NOODLE BOWL

Who doesn't love a noodle bowl? Zippy and fresh, this noodle bowl comes together quickly and is sure to please everyone's palate. Don't let all the ingredients scare you! With a little chopping, you can pull this recipe together faster than you can get takeout. Please read through the instructions first so that you will understand the quick flow of your oriental noodle bowl. This recipe makes two large bowls.

INGREDIENTS:
For the meat and marinade:
   A little less than one pound chicken or steak
   1 large clove of garlic (smashed and minced)
   ½ tablespoon peeled, grated fresh ginger
   2 tablespoons soy sauce
   ¼ teaspoon red pepper flakes
   1 tablespoon olive oil
   2 tablespoons chia gel

For the salad:
   2 to 3 large handfuls of spinach or salad greens of your choice
   ½ cucumber (deseeded and chopped)
   1 small carrot (julienne-sliced)
   1 handful fresh cilantro (stems removed and chopped)
   2 radishes (thinly sliced)

¼ round of red onion (minced)

1 small handful of broccoli slaw (available in pouches)

1 teaspoon dried mint

2 packages ramen noodles (with the package of seasoning discarded)

Peanuts or sunflower seeds for garnish, if desired

FOR THE SALAD DRESSING:

½ tablespoon peeled, grated fresh ginger

1 teaspoon agave or honey

2 tablespoons rice wine vinegar or apple vinegar

A couple of grinds of fresh black pepper

1 tablespoon olive oil

INSTRUCTIONS:

FOR THE MEAT AND MARINADE:

Place all the ingredients into a pie pan (or flat pan) and stir with a fork. Place your thinly cut steak strips (which can be grilled leftovers) or chicken strips into the marinade for about ten minutes, turning once. We often just use meat as a flavor garnish—you be the judge of the quantity you would like to use.

FOR THE SALAD AND DRESSING:

While the meat marinates, prepare your veggies and place them into a large bowl. Begin boiling the water for the ramen noodles. Remove the ramen from its packet and break the noodle square into quarters and throw away the foil packet. Pour the meat and marinade into a small, preheated skillet and sauté. Cook until the chicken is no longer pink or the beef is cooked to your liking. Remove the skillet from heat and set aside the meat, leaving only the marinade in the skillet.

Add the ramen noodles to the boiling water and cook as directed on the package.

Wisk together all ingredients for the salad dressing and pour them over the veggie salad bowl. Toss to coat.

Now that the ramen is cooked, drain the noodles and toss them into the skillet with the marinade to coat.

To assemble your noodle bowls, place noodles on the bottom, add the veggies and then the meat, and garnish with peanuts or seeds of choice. Some of us at the MySeeds Chia Test Kitchen would starve if we had to use chopsticks to eat our noodle bowls. Are you up to the challenge? We require forks—darn more practice!

QUINOA AND CHIA BLACK BEAN SALAD

Here's a satisfying salad that's high in protein. Because this salad is loaded with protein and fiber from the quinoa and chia, you'll feel full faster. It is low in carbohydrates, but you'll feel satisfied anyway. The southwest flavorings blend together with the veggies to create a wonderfully robust, satisfying meal—fast and easy. If you add a small, grilled, spicy chicken breast on the side, we're sure you will say, "Olé"! This recipe makes two servings but is easily doubled because it is great cold too.

INGREDIENTS:
   ¼ cup quinoa
   1 tablespoon dry chia
   ⅔ cup vegetable broth
   2 slices of red onion, diced
   ½ 15-oz can black beans, rinsed
   ⅓ cup frozen or fresh corn
   Small sweet yellow pepper, diced
   1 tablespoon olive oil
   ½ teaspoon ground cumin
   ⅛ teaspoon cayenne pepper
   2 handfuls dark salad greens of your choice

Fresh diced tomato

½ an avocado, sliced or diced

INSTRUCTIONS:

In a skillet that has a lid, sauté the onion in the small amount of oil. Remove the skillet from the heat and pour in the veggie broth, quinoa, and chia. Stir to combine. Return to a much lower heat setting and cover. Prepare the black beans, dice the pepper, and measure the amount of corn. Add these ingredients and stir to combine. Re-cover with the lid. The absorption of the liquid by the quinoa and chia should take about another ten minutes, but do check it occasionally. Prepare your greens, tomato, and avocado condiments for the top of your salad. Plate with a greenery foundation, then add the quinoa and place the condiments on top. "Muy fácil y bien."

Note: We wanted to add a jicama, but, darn, they were out of season. This root has a crisp, light flavor that is loaded with fiber. In addition to vitamin C, jicama also contains smaller amount of important vitamins and minerals such as magnesium, vitamin E, and iron.

CHIA PESTO BURGER

Craving a different burger rather than the old standard of lettuce, tomato, and mayo? Check out this spinach-basil pesto burger! This is a super burger with less meat. This pesto is great on both beef and leaner turkey burgers. You will be entering a whole new dimension when you try this alternative topping. It is easy to add a new twist to backyard grilling or to your inside grill. Are you inviting super health-conscious friends over? Try this very lean burger recipe too! This recipe will make about one-half cup of pesto.

INGREDIENTS:

2 cups fresh spinach leaves (with large stems removed)

½ cup basil leaves (if you are short on fresh basil, you can augment with dried, using less, of course)

2 to 4 tablespoons parmesan cheese

2 cloves garlic

2 to 3 tablespoons olive oil

1 tablespoon chia seeds

INSTRUCTIONS:

Place all the ingredients into your mini chopper and chop into a fine paste. Begin by using two tablespoons of olive oil; however, you may need just a little more to incorporate all the elements. Now you're ready to make the burger listed below.

BASIL CHIA BEAN BURGER

These tasty turkey burgers have black beans mixed right in. These burgers not only taste great but also include more fiber and lead you to use less meat. With the pesto you made in the recipe above, you have a great burger alternative. These should be grilled indoors or on foil on your outdoor grill. You can serve these with a nice slice of mozzarella cheese. This recipe makes three to four burgers.

INGREDIENTS:

½ pound ground turkey

½ of a 15-oz can black beans, rinsed and smashed

8 basil leaves (or 1 tablespoon dried basil)

2 tablespoons dry chia seeds

1 egg

2 tablespoons bread crumbs

1 slice of mozzarella cheese (optional)

INSTRUCTIONS:

In a bowl, place the black beans and smash them with the back of a fork to create a very chunky paste. Add the ground turkey, basil, chia, egg, and bread crumbs. With your hands, mix the ingredients so that they are all evenly distributed throughout. Form into patties and let them rest so that the chia absorbs any excess moisture. Broil or grill about four minutes per side. While the burgers are still warm, add the pesto and the slice of cheese. Press the bun down and you're ready to serve.

GLUTEN-FREE PEANUT BUTTER BANANA COOKIES

A friend of ours has been making these for years and we *love* them. Chia works great in your gluten-free recipes! These little cookie balls have only fruit sugar (no added sugars or HFCS). We believe that cookies are good for the soul, once in a while. So, the next time you want to stir up a quick treat, why not make it just a little bit healthier?

INGREDIENTS:

> 3 medium ripe bananas, smashed
> 2 cups quick-cooking oats
> ¼ cup unsweetened cocoa powder
> ¼ cup unsweetened natural peanut butter, stirred if separated
> 1 tablespoon dry chia
> ⅓ cup unsweetened applesauce
> 1 teaspoon vanilla

INSTRUCTIONS:

In a medium bowl smash the bananas to a small but chunky consistency. Dump the oats, cocoa powder, and chia on top of the smashed bananas. Add the peanut butter. (Note: For the most "peanutty" taste in your baking, it is wise to use all-natural peanut butter. Natural peanut butter is also better for you; it has no added sugars or high fructose corn syrup.)

Add the applesauce and the vanilla. The batter will seem very dry at first, but it *will* all combine. Let the batter rest for about ten minutes while the chia absorbs any extra moisture. Drop by the teaspoonful (we use the convenient cookie scoop utensil) and bake at 350 degrees Fahrenheit on a cookie sheet coated with cooking spray for about ten to twelve minutes. The bottom of the cookies should be lightly browned when done. This recipe makes a little over two dozen cookies. Once the cookies have cooled, place in an airtight container. These cookies also freeze well.

INTENSELY CHOCOLATE CHIA BROWNIES

When you *need* a chocolate fix, you don't need all the sugar and fat, you just crave chocolate. Can you bake with a natural sugar substitute in the My Seeds Chia Test Kitchen recipes? You bet! These easy brownies bake in about twenty minutes and give you the chocolate you require. If you get a serious craving, you may as well just give into it with a little bite or portion-controlled helping so that you are not preoccupied by the thought and then feel deprived and overindulge at a later time. These brownies can be your answer. Be thoughtful, but enjoy the experience!

INGREDIENTS:
   ½ cup flour
   ⅓ cup unsweetened cocoa powder
   ¼ teaspoon baking powder
   Dash salt
   ¼ cup vegetable oil
   ¼ cup chia gel
   2 eggs
   ½ cup sugar
   ½ cup sugar substitute such as stevia (if in packets, use 12)
   1 teaspoon vanilla
   ½ cup chocolate chips or nuts of your choice

INSTRUCTIONS:

In small bowl combine the flour, cocoa powder, baking powder, and salt. Stir to combine. In a second bowl, place the vegetable oil, chia gel, sugar, sugar substitute, eggs, and vanilla. Next, stir the wet ingredients together to thoroughly incorporate the eggs. Slowly add the dry ingredients. Stir in the nuts or chocolate chips. Pour into a baking pan coated with cooking spray and bake at 350 degrees Fahrenheit for about twenty to twenty-five minutes. Cool before cutting into squares.

Chia Seed FAQ

Want quick answers to your top chia questions? Look no further than this handy FAQ. The various chapters of the book elaborate on many of the points you can find here, but if you want to get started right away, this is the place to be.

Q: Do I have to do anything to chia seeds before I eat them?

A: It depends on how you want to use your chia. You don't have to do anything if you just want to sprinkle the seeds on foods such as baked potatoes, salads, yogurts, ice cream, or soup. It's as easy as scoop, sprinkle, and eat. There's no messy grinding.

Note: Do not attempt to wash chia seeds. They will immediately become sticky and start absorbing the water to form chia gel.

If you're using chia seeds as a fat substitute in your recipes, you have to make the gel first. Use our easy, free gel recipe (in this book), and in fifteen minutes you're ready to use them to replace one-third of the fat in your recipes, without reducing any of the flavors. The gel can be made ahead of time and keeps up to two weeks in the fridge in a covered container.

Q: When is the best time to eat chia seeds?
A: The best time depends on why you are using them.

If you want to stay hydrated longer, eat them before a workout or playing sports, with a bottle of water or sports drink. You can mix them into the drink, or consume a dry tablespoon then drink the liquid right away to hydrate the seeds.

To curb appetite and improve regularity, eat chia seeds in the morning or right before meals.

Q: How much chia should I eat in one day?
A: That depends on how you are using it. For general purposes of health, nutrition, and energy, an adult would usually consume about one tablespoon of dry seeds (or nine tablespoons of gelled seeds) in one day. Every bag of MySeeds Chia has more than thirty servings, so it will last more than one month, costing less than $1 per day to use. However, if you are using the seeds to fight hunger or stay feeling full longer, you can, of course, use more. Chia is extremely safe. Only you know when you're feeling full, so let your body tell you the amount that's right for you.

Q: How should I store my chia seeds?
A: Chia seeds do not require refrigeration or any special storage container. As long as you keep the bag in a dry place your seeds will stay fresh and ready to use. Chia has an exceptionally long shelf life because of its high antioxidant content.

Chia gel will keep in a covered container in the refrigerator for up to two weeks.

Q: How long before chia seeds generally expire?
A: Because of their high level of antioxidants, chia seeds of any color will not go rancid like flax seed or other

oils and grains will. They will keep safely for up to two years! Their antioxidant content prevents the oils from spoiling and also helps you prevent oxidation in your body's cells when you consume them.

Q: What does chia taste like?

A: Any color of chia seeds have very little flavor. Adding them to food will not change the taste of the food. If eaten plain, or as an unflavored gel, there is a vague, almost nut-like taste. Because there's so little flavor to chia seeds, it's almost impossible to hate them.

Note: If making chia gel, always use filtered or bottled water. Because the seeds distribute flavors, using tap water could adversely affect the flavor of your gel.

Q: How can chia seeds make my recipes better?

A: When used as a gel in cooking, chia seeds do not absorb flavors, they distribute flavors. This means that you can use them to replace the volume of foods without cutting back on taste. If you substitute one-third of a recipe's fat (where a recipe requires something such as butter, shortening, or margarine) with chia gel, the finished food will taste the same, but have one-third less fat. Of course, you are also adding all the healthy benefits of chia seeds, such as vitamins, antioxidants, and calcium, to the food.

Q: Can I use chia gel to replace the volume of fatty foods?

A: Yes! If you enjoy the taste of salad dressings, BBQ sauce, or any number of other condiments but wish you didn't have to deal with the calorie and fat content they add, chia is the answer.

Chia seeds do not absorb flavors; they distribute flavors. The seeds do not alter the taste of the food or drink you add them to.

They don't take away flavors from your foods or drinks. You can use them to replace the volume of foods without cutting back on taste. This also helps you cut down on the amount of food you eat. For instance, if you love the taste of a salad dressing, but wish it didn't add calories to your healthy salad, you can mix in chia gel. A little bit of dressing will now cover your whole salad, and taste the same as if you had used the full amount of dressing.

Q: Are chia seeds in general approved by the FDA?

A: Yes, chia seeds are classified by the FDA as a healthy food.

Q: Are pesticides used on chia seeds?

A: Generally, no pesticides are used on chia. Pesticides are not needed because the plant contains a special oil in the leaves and stems. Insects and other pests won't attack or try to eat the plants because they can't stand the oil. If chia is being grown in a natural, native environment, it won't need any pesticides, chemical fertilizers, or other unnatural additions. It's a super safe crop!

Q: Do I have to give up eating anything to eat chia seeds?

A: Not really! You can supplement whatever you are already eating with chia. In fact, we encourage you to use the seeds on foods you already like. The benefit of chia occurs when each seed absorbs nine times its weight in water and forms a nutritious gel. The gel fills you up, so you shouldn't feel like snacking or over-eating at mealtime.

Q: Is chia fortified with any vitamins or pharmaceuticals?

A: Chia seeds are so healthy already in their natural state that any tinkering isn't necessary. They're full of vitamins, minerals, and antioxidants as well as natural essential oils (e.g., omega-3), protein, and fiber. They don't require additives, as they are already a super-healthy food. Their high level of antioxidants acts as a natural preservative, keeping them fresh for up to two years if stored in a dry place. MySeeds chia is 100 percent natural with no additives or preservatives.

Q: Will chia help with regularity?

A: Yes! Chia seeds contain eleven grams of fiber, so you're getting 44 percent of your daily value in just one ounce. They help retain water throughout the digestive process, keeping your digestive tract hydrated and clean. These two factors combine to greatly aid in regularity and digestion.

The soluble fiber in chia seeds may help lower your cholesterol as well.

"Clinical studies show that a heart-healthy diet (low in saturated fat and cholesterol, and high in fruits, vegetables, and grain products that contain soluble fiber) can lower blood cholesterol. In these studies, cholesterol levels dropped between 0.5 percent and 2 percent for every gram of soluble fiber eaten per day."[57]

The soluble fiber also stabilizes blood sugar by slowing the release of carbohydrates in the digestive system.

Q: What happens if I eat more than the recommended amount in a day?

A: There is no set daily amount. If you become hungry and want to use more seed to avoid unhealthy snacks, you can. Your body will tell you what's the right amount for you.

---

57   "Using the Nutrition Facts Label: A Guide for Older Adults" www.fda.gov/downloads/Food/IngredientsPackagingLabeling/UCM275396.pdf (Accessed June 2013)

Q: What happens if my pet eats my chia seeds?

A: Chia should not hurt your pet dog, cat, bird, or rodent. Chia seeds are healthy for anyone. The omega-3 and -6 oils in the seeds help build strong, shiny coats. If your pets eat an excessive amount of seeds, they may become very thirsty, so be sure they have access to plenty of water.

Q: Are chia seeds gluten- and cholesterol-free? I heard they have oils inside.

A: Yes! Chia provides you with a balance of omega-3 (alpha-linolenic acid) and omega-6 (linoleic acid). It's actually the best plant-based source of healthy omega-3 available. Unlike fish and fish oils, chia delivers all this healthy oil without any cholesterol. With all-natural chia as your source of omega-3, you won't need to worry about heavy metals that can be found in some fish.

Unlike other grains, chia is free of gluten. Antioxidants that occur naturally in chia keep these oils from going rancid.

Q: Will chia seeds force me to lose weight if I just want to eat them for their nutritional value and other health benefits (colon hydration, blood sugar balancing, diabetes, protein, etc.)?

A: No, eating chia will not force you to lose weight if you are not eating it in the predetermined "weight loss ways." Chia can be used in two ways: first, for losing weight, and, second, for maintaining health and improving nutrition. All you'll need to do is avoid the weight-loss methods, which include the following:

1. Eating lots of chia right before meals so as to fill up and not eat as much as you would have otherwise.

2. Mixing higher amounts of chia into foods so that the food fills you up faster and makes you eat less of it.

3. Using chia in a bottle of juice or water to fill up and avoid snacking or using this method to skip meals. (In this case, you would want to reach for a healthy snack instead, such as granola or fruit.)

Basically, if you're not using chia to avoid food or eat less food than you normally would or just using chia by itself to fill up or skip mealtimes, it's not going to make you lose weight. It does have complete protein and omega-3 oils which are important in maintaining a healthy weight. Our recipes use a moderate amount (that's adjustable, in most cases) for butter, oil, and fat replacement, flavor enhancement, and general nutrition.

> Q: What do doctors say about eating seeds with diverticulitis or diverticulosis?
>
> A: Different doctors may say slightly different things. The bottom line seems to be that avoiding all seeds and nuts is no longer the mainstream advice. You should certainly read the helpful doctors' quotes below to learn more about what they have to say. (This book is not written by a doctor, but the quotes are by real MDs and the study cited below was conducted and written up by the US government.)

Of course, the key thing to remember is that everyone *is* different and everyone's condition will vary. Consult *your* doctor about your own condition and your own specific needs, and, remember, if it bothers you, don't do it! Ultimately, you are the one in charge of your own diet and health practices. Doing what works best for your own personal health is the key.

> Q: What do doctors say about the use of seeds with diverticulitis?
>
> A: The following are quotes from actual doctors regarding the use of seeds with this condition. As usual, before

taking on any diet change for health or weight loss, you should ask your doctor to determine the best approach for your own specific needs. You can learn more from each doctor by searching for his name on the Internet.

Michael Picco, MD (from the Mayo Clinic)[58] has this to say: "In the past, many doctors recommended that people with diverticulosis avoid seeds and nuts, including foods with small seeds, such as tomatoes, cucumbers, and strawberries. It was thought that these tiny particles could lodge in the diverticula and cause inflammation (diverticulitis). But there is no scientific evidence that seeds and nuts cause diverticulitis flares. In fact, eating a high-fiber diet—which may include nuts and seeds—may reduce the risk of diverticular disease."

Andrew Weil, MD[59] (author of several health books and a website), says, "I think it's fine to experiment with some seeds or nuts to find out whether or how much you can tolerate these foods. Another important strategy to prevent an attack is to add other types of fiber to your diet in the form of wheat bran or psyllium. You can buy powdered psyllium seed husks at health food stores without the sweeteners and dyes found in drugstore products. Be sure to drink plenty of water when you're taking these bulking agents. You also may feel better during diverticulitis attacks if you take a stool softener such as Dialose, Colace, or another brand containing docusate, a drug that is available over the counter. Try to relieve stress through deep breathing exercises, yoga, or other stress-reduction methods. In the past,[60] many doctors recommended that people with diverticulosis avoid foods

58   Michael Picco, MD, Mayo Clinic Q & A, http://www.mayoclinic.com/health/diverticulitis-diet/AN01255 (Accessed 20 October 2013)

59   Dr. Andrew Weil, MD, Library, http://www.drweil.com/drw/u/id/QAA26673 (Accessed 20 October 2013)

60   Dr. Andrew Weil, MD, Library "Diverticulitis Dilemma," http://www.drweil.com/drw/u/QAA400945/Diverticulitis-Dilemma.html (Accessed 20 October 2013)

with small seeds such as tomatoes or strawberries, because they believed that the particles could lodge in the diverticula and cause inflammation. While there's no evidence supporting this idea, some people do find that eating nuts and seeds during an attack of diverticulitis can be irritating to the inflamed intestinal lining, so for them I would suggest staying away from them."

Timothy Harlan, MD (also known as Dr. Gourmet),[61] says, "In the past there has been some controversy about the treatment of this problem, with many doctors telling their patients with diverticulosis to not eat popcorn, seeds, nuts, or foods that contain seeds, such as those found in tomatoes, cucumbers, and strawberries. In the past there was never any solid research to support this, however. In the last few years good studies have disproved that a problem exists.

"I have always thought the theory a bit silly but almost certainly so with strawberry seeds (those things are tiny!). Guidelines no longer make this recommendation, and I do not for my patients. The studies have shown that the only dietary change that will make a difference for those with diverticulosis is a high-fiber diet (and, of course, a high-fiber diet is the recommendation for all of us).

"One of the largest studies on this subject was published on September 8, 2008. Researchers looked at more than 47,000 men over eighteen years of age as part of the Health Professionals Follow-up Study. The most fascinating finding was that those men who ate the most nuts and popcorn actually had lower risk of infection. In short, no association was found between an increased risk of diverticulitis and eating nuts, popcorn, or corn (JAMA 2008;300(8):907–914)."

The US government also weighs in on the issue on this web page: digestive.niddk.nih.gov/ddiseases/pubs/diverticulosis/.

61　Timothy Harlan, "Diverticulitis Nuts & Seeds," Dr. Gourmet, http://www.drgourmet.com/column/dr/2008/090808.shtml#.UmcNKMXD-bg

Note: All quotes and studies were created by, and belong to, their original authors.

Q: Where do MySeeds chia seeds come from?

MySeeds chia seeds are grown in Mexico. Our chia is from the western side of Mexico where the soil is sandy and dry. These aren't ideal growing conditions for other crops, but they're great for chia seeds. Mexico is where chia seeds were discovered (though they will grow elsewhere). Chia seeds are thought to be named for the Chiapas Region where they were discovered.

CONCLUSION

We hope you have enjoyed this chia book! Now you know all the currently studied ways the chia seed can help you in various aspects of your life. This super seed is just so versatile, helpful, and easy to use that you'll never run out of ways to use it, or reasons to use it.

Remember that there are no quick fixes for most health-related issues. Healthy eating and exercise are the ultimate keys to real health improvement, now and over the long term. Now that you know some of the pitfalls of the modern, available foods (companies trying to create food addictions on purpose, the chemicals that can sabotage your health, etc.), you're more prepared to use chia to make the changes you want to see. As for weight loss, there's too much focus on losing as much weight as you can over the shortest period of time. It's popular because everyone wants a quick fix and instant results or they don't think whatever they are currently doing is working. But remember that your focus should be on how you want to live your life one year from now or even twenty-five years from now. What are you going to be doing then? How are you going to be feeling at that time? It has to be fun, it has to be delicious, and it has to be something easy enough that you can do it every day. Health is something you achieve each day, not a deprivation period you can go through for a couple of weeks and then be done with it.

Chia is something you can easily use in the long term, because of its lack of flavor. You can't get tired of it because you can't even tell it's in most foods. Variety, ease of use, and not having to add another expense to your life are key points in being able to continue a new habit into the future. Chia isn't expensive and you can actually save money in the long term by eating fresh and smart by making food at home.

If you liked these chia recipes, you might want more! We've got a whole cookbook full of *just* chia recipes for you to enjoy. It's the *Chia Seed Cookbook* by the MySeeds Chia Test Kitchen. It has 224 pages of recipes, with all full-color photos, so that you can see exactly what you can make. Each recipe in this present book is here to help illustrate a point, whether it is how chia can cut the fat in baked goods, or to prove that chia works in your low-sugar recipes too. With a cookbook dedicated to only recipes of every type, you can make chia breakfasts, lunches, dinners, appetizers, and desserts. The recipes there are also for everyday cooks and busy people who still want something healthier on their plate.

You can learn more about or get this book at www.mychiaseeds.com/CookBook/TheChiaSeedCookBook.html, which has a link to where the book is listed on Amazon.com.

If you want to see video demos of recipes, you can go to www.mychiaseeds.com to watch chia in action, demonstrated for you. Chia is so much fun to experiment with and so easy to use that you'll wonder why you didn't discover it earlier! Now that you know so much more about chia seeds, you can get started using them right away. Enjoy your healthier life!

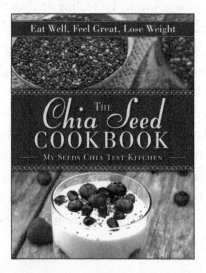

INDEX

· · · · ·